Infertility
On The
Internet

How To Get On-Line
And In Charge Of Your Fertility

by Julie Watson

Infertility On The Internet

How To Get On-Line And In Charge Of Your Fertility

Julie Watson

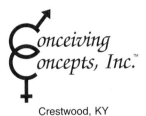

Conceiving Concepts, Inc.™

Crestwood, KY

Check us, and the Author's story, out on the Web at
www.conceivingconcepts.com

First Printing 1997

ISBN 0-9660816-1-7

Edited by Corinne Greenberg
Cover and book design by GetSET, Crestwood, KY

Library of Congress Catalog Card Number 97-77145

Watson, Julie

Infertility on the Internet: How to Get On-Line
and In Charge of Your Fertility/
Julie Watson - First edition.

A portion of the profits from this and all publications of Conceiving Concepts, Inc. will be donated to our Fertility Foundation to help those who cannot afford fertility treatments.

ATTENTION ASSOCIATIONS AND ORGANIZATIONS: Quantity discounts are available on bulk purchases of this book. For information please contact the publisher at Conceiving Concepts, Inc. P.O. Box 869, Crestwood, KY 40014 (502) 241-8497.

To my husband, Matthew,
whose steadfast love got me through our infertility experience
and made this all possible.
I love you!

ACKNOWLEDGEMENTS

Obviously, this book would not have become a reality without my ride on the infertility rollercoaster. Although the experience has been a total nightmare at times, I would like to thank several people for getting me through it and giving me the inspiration to write this book.

I would first like thank my mom and dad for inspiring me to write this book in the first place (and for giving me the many tools to do it)!

I would also like to thank the many friends who are also in our shoes, for their helpful and loving support, as well as our countless other fertile friends who have been so remarkably sensitive to our situation.

I especially want to thank Dr. Donald Cline and his staff for their utmost, courteous patient care throughout our fertility treatments.

And finally, most of all, I wish to thank our Lord — for giving me so many gifts, too numerous to count.

TABLE OF CONTENTS

FOREWORD

The need for a team approach to infertility is very important. Cooperation and understanding between the infertile couple, their extended families, peers, employers, clergy, and the medical care givers may make a difference in success, and certainly will make a difference in attitudes.

Infertility on the Internet offers another resource for those who wish to be active in the diagnosis/treatment/resolution process faced by all infertile couples. Julie Watson has had more than a casual interest in infertility over the last several years. Her continued interest, study and experience are manifested in this presentation. She has interwoven her personal experience with infertility and the Internet, as is only possible for a person knowledgeable in both areas. The amount of research required to construct this volume has been monumental. Trying to compile a complete and comprehensive guide to sites on the Internet in relation to infertility (while many of these sites are either "getting on or getting off the information superhighway") is certainly a formidable task. The author has not only succeeded in doing that very thing, but has been able to categorize and explain the sites so that they can be used by the most novice or the most experienced "surfer."

However, a word of warning: although this book is extremely well written, factual and accurate as it explains the Internet resource, the actual Internet sites may not always be well written, factual or accurate. As the author will warn you as well, information obtained from the Internet should *always* be subject to a "second opinion."

The reader will not be disappointed with this volume. The availability of a complete, comprehensive, well organized, and well reasoned review of Internet resources has been needed for some time. The author has provided this in a personal and professional manner.

Donald L. Cline, MD
Associate Clinical Professor of Obstetrics and Gynecology
Indiana University School of Medicine
Indianapolis, IN

INTRODUCTION

WHY YOU NEED TO SURF THE NET
(And Words of Advice from Someone Who's "Been There")

The old cliché "knowledge is power" is more than appropriate in a couple's battle with infertility — it is *imperative*. After emotionally struggling through months, and often years, of what seems to be endless tests and failed treatment attempts, couples often seem to reach a state of helplessness and become trapped by their situation. They begin to feel as if there is nothing that they can do. They feel out of control. However, there is power a couple can attain in this situation. And that is the power of knowledge. Knowledge that can be obtained and used — to find the right doctor, to cope with their situation, and to identify treatments which suit their particular emotional, ethical, and financial needs. Knowledge is what gives a couple back what they think they might have lost (and the most valuable weapon in this battle) — control. Control once again over their situation and a renewed sense of hope that they, too, can win this war.

But where do you find this knowledge? More and more books, technical articles and journals continue to be published regarding all aspects of infertility — from the emotional side, to choosing a right doctor, to discussion of causes, to the various treatment methods available. Although many of the books are a "must read" for anyone experiencing infertility, they are still sometimes hard to find and are limited in scope. Journals and technical articles are also helpful, but most of the time these are even harder to find or their availability may be unknown to battling couples. Such resources have been hard to find until now — the wonderful age of the Internet, the most valuable up-to-date tool available to all couples in their battle over infertility.

In our 7-year quest for a child, we wasted so much precious time doing nothing — a state many infertiles refer to as "denial." Time would heal us. However, month after month, the "next month it will happen" never came. Looking back with the hindsight we now have, there are several bits of advice I would give anyone who suspects they may have a fertility problem; or anyone struggling with infertility for some time. Mind you, everything I say here is not advice my husband and I used from day one. (In fact we never got much advice from anyone who was battling infertility. The only advice we ever seemed to get was from a well-meaning, but clueless, fertile world.) No, we did it the hard way and had to learn from our mistakes. But I hope with this advice — and by use of this book — a few more couples will be spared some of the hurt infertility can afflict upon a couple. Therefore, these are my four suggestions on how to wage the war with the least amount of casualties:

- **FIND A REPUTABLE INFERTILITY SPECIALIST!** First and foremost, I cannot emphasize this advice enough. Do not waste your time on seeing your regular OB/GYN — especially if treating female problems and delivering babies is their primary line of business. Some OBs have the infertility credentials, but you must find out what those credentials are in order to know that you are in good hands and that they are not wasting your time. Many other books (and also selected web sites discussed in this book) can provide the needed advice on how to choose and work with your infertility specialist. This then leads my second bit of advice:

- **READ!** Read, read, and read some more. Educate yourself with anything and everything you can get your hands on regarding infertility and increasing your fertility. I never enjoyed reading much beyond the Sunday comics. But, as I began to accept our situation and face the fact that we might have a problem, I began trying to find a solution to "fix" the situation, and reading gave me that tool. Always remember — knowledge is your main weapon in this battle! With time you will find that the more you read, the easier you will be able to decipher your own body's signals and your own situation. Nothing can substitute for excellent medical care. But what complements excellent medical care is a patient with a firm understanding of *what* is being tested, *why* is it being tested, and what the results *really* mean.

Even the best reproductive physicians may be unable to always answer these questions for each couple. *It is the duty of the couple then, to make sure that they have a firm understanding of their treatment* and the logical progression of the series of tests which will be administered to them. Infertility now affects one out of every six couples — which some call an epidemic. But, although the statistics look grim, our generation of doctors now know more than ever about the causes of infertility, and they are ever developing ways of helping couples achieve conception. Still, these physicians have limited office hours and often carry large patient loads — possibly due to the high patient-demand / physician-supply ratio. Needless to say, many infertility patients do not feel as if they get their diagnosis and treatments thoroughly explained to them, let alone get the emotional support they so desperately need in this delicate situation. Having said that, the third suggestion is:

- **QUESTION!** When you do not understand a prescribed treatment, or if your doctor is going faster or slower with your treatment than you'd like — *question*. If you find information in your reading that contradicts what your doctor may be telling you — *question*. Question him or her about your treatment. And *don't feel intimidated about doing it!* Remember, it's part of their job to answer your questions. If the answers you are getting do not "feel" right to you, that is, if the type or progression of treatment he or she wants to administer does not seem logical to you — then it might be time to reevaluate your doctor's objectives with your own. If you don't believe or understand what I'm saying then check out the details of how we almost got burnt by our first reproductive specialist during our fertility battle. You can read our long gory story on the publisher's page at www.conceivingconcepts.com. Believe me, we almost had to learn this one lesson the hard way. Finally, and probably most importantly:

- **GET SUPPORT!** Whether it's from a support group support such as RESOLVE, a friend who has also gone through infertility, or whether you use any of the wonderful support mechanisms available on the Web — get support! We fought our battle WAY too long without it. The lack of it almost cost us not only our sanity, but our marriage as well. Realize that getting support is not a sign of weakness. It is way or regaining control — control over your emotions — something that infertility quickly robs from you.

Enough said and enough advice given. You have purchased this book to aid in your quest for knowledge. And that we will do. This book is meant to help not only the beginners, but also those already familiar with the Internet. So pull your chair up to your computer, plug in your modem, and let's get started on our journey. What? You don't have a computer? Never fear — read on anyway! Once you see for yourself what wonderful resources are available on the Internet then you WILL find someway to access it. I assure you. You will not want to miss out on this!

CHAPTER 1
GETTING STARTED ON THE INTERNET

Understanding the Net and All that It Offers

I was doing more obsessing today, and I realized what bad shape I'd be in if it wasn't for the Net.

There is all of the support from all the wonderful people out there.

There is all of the useful information there, when I need it.

But it goes deeper than that—

Without the Net I'd be going into my doctor's appointments with little to no idea what was going to happen, a situation that makes me very uncomfortable.

I got my recommendation for my doctor from someone I met on the Net. I knew what to ask for when I first called to set up the meeting.

The books I have are largely ones that have been recommended by the various web sites. I also know enough to ignore some of the crazier books that have some downright scary information in them.

I knew what the insurance situation was going to be like, so I'm not surprised when problems come up.

So, 3 cheers for the Net!

Laura —From the ONNA Mailing List

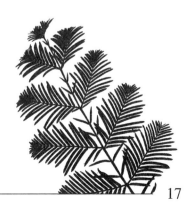

Surely upon finding this book you must have thought the title of it to be odd. After all, how could something as personal as infertility be tied to something so popular and exposed as the Internet? So, before we hit the specifics of *what* the Internet is and *how* to use it, let's look at *why* the Internet can become your best asset if you are struggling with fertility problems.

WHY THE INTERNET?

As you can see from the quote at the beginning of this chapter, the reasons to use the Internet to get through your infertility battle are vast. In the field of reproduction, technical advancements are made daily. For this reason, it is difficult and possibly foolish to completely rely on "old" technical information laid out in printed media alone. On the other hand, the Internet is alive! It provides a forum where the most *up-to-date* information on all subjects may be found. (In fact, the Internet was actually first used by universities as a way of housing research documents.) Therefore, the Internet provides a couple struggling with infertility information on the best diagnostic evaluation and latest advancements in treatments.

In addition, the Internet allows access to very specific and sometimes hard to find information. Take for example that you want to find out which states mandate insurance coverage for infertility treatment. Is your state one of them? Once you learn how to accurately search the Internet, you will be just a few keystrokes away from finding specific information that you need. For instance, you can not only find out if insurance coverage is mandated in your state, but also, if it is not, you may learn ways of how you can fight for coverage.

Some of the various tools on the Internet, such as mailing lists, bulletin boards, and chat rooms allow you to gain another invaluable resource — support. You can find and converse with individuals who are also battling infertility, with the added bonus of *anonymity.* By using these tools to share similar stories, compare diagnosis, and treatments, you will no longer feel alone! It's quite comforting to be able to lay out your feelings on the keyboard while being able to hide in the shelter of cyberspace. I also feel that just the process of putting your emotions and feelings into words is therapeutic.

Lastly, the best and most defining asset that the Internet offers is that it's fun to use! Sad to say, many folks do not like to read, even if reading self-help books provides some peace of mind and will help them in their struggle. I have known many people battling infertility who have never cracked a book to get information that would help them! However, once I show them what the Internet offers and how to use it, they are hooked.

FOR BEGINNERS:
WHAT THE INTERNET IS & HOW TO GET STARTED

Keep in mind that this chapter's main purpose is to get you started — to give you the minimal amount of tools to get around the Internet and access the information which you need as it relates to infertility. Anymore, there are literally hundreds of books written on how to use the Internet. I have included some of the very easiest of these books to read in the Suggested Reading section at the back of this book, should you wish to explore more of its features which are not covered in this short chapter and to familiarize yourself more with computer terminology. For those of you who have already been on the Internet, you may want to quickly skim through the rest of this chapter, to pick up any new tips, and then move quickly onto the next chapter.

WHAT IS THE INTERNET?

The Internet is simply a vast array of interlinked computers. No particular entity owns the whole thing. This concept of interlinking computers (and thus the birth of the Internet) originated during the cold war when the government created it as a safe haven for important document transfer. Since then, it has grown and been used for many years by universities to share research articles, software programs, and other pertinent information. However, the software used to connect the vast array of computers was crude and not very "user-friendly."

Then came the dawn of the World Wide Web. The Web, as it is commonly called, and the Internet are not one and the same, although many people mistake them to be. The Web was the catalyst, however, which made the Internet usable for the first time to the general public. The Web uses a friendlier software system that transforms the boring text documents on the Internet with color, sound, animation and pizzazz. The Web does this by using a communications software known as HTTP (short for Hypertext Transfer Protocol) which allows documents to be standardized so that they then may be easily shared between different computers. Because of this, HTTP allows documents to easily be accessed or "linked" to other documents.

If you look at a Web page you will often see words which are colored and/or underlined. These are the links (also known as hyperlinks, or Hot Buttons) to other Web pages. An author of one Web page can thus link his page to another page he created (or any of the other million Web pages available on the Internet) because of HTTP. Please note, however, that hyperlinks are not always displayed as underlined words on a page, but also can be accessed by the viewer by clicking on the pictures (also known as icons or buttons) on the Web page. The designer of the page makes that decision. When viewing a Web page, make sure not to overlook icons which may lead you to other Web pages.

But what makes up a Web page? Simply, it is text enhanced with sounds, animation, and colored graphics which a person creates. It usually is formatted in the software language known as HTML (Hypertext Markup Language.) After a Web page is created using HTML, it then resides on one of the computers on the Internet and then can be accessed by the HTTP which the Web uses. Got all that? I know it's confusing but, unless you are going to develop your own Web page, it really is not all that necessary for you to know if you are just going to *use* the Internet.

WHAT ABOUT E-MAIL, NEWSGROUPS, CHAT FORUMS, FTP, GOPHER — AREN'T THOSE PART OF THE INTERNET TOO?

Yes, as we previously mentioned the Web is *not* the only system which resides on the Internet. Perhaps the first system which was universally used before the Web was electronic mail (e-mail). As with the Web, e-mail uses software to direct its messages from one computer system to another. In fact, as you will learn in Chapter 5, e-mail was one of the first systems that people utilized to share information regarding infertility. Mailing lists, which use e-mail systems to distribute messages to large groups of individuals, still remain a primary support mechanism for some people.

As we will learn more in Chapter 5, Newgroups and Chat Rooms are also independent systems which run on the Internet. Newgroups and Bulletin Boards are very similar and provide a public place in cyberspace to post and respond to messages. Chat Rooms basically are systems which have the ability to provide on-line real-time conversation.

Some of the older systems which were used in the "dark ages" of the Internet still exist today. It could be said that FTP (file transfer protocol) is somewhat analogous to what HTTP is today. However, where FTP only has the capability of transfering files, HTTP has the capability of organizing not only text files, but graphic and sound files and constructing them into what we see as Web pages. GOPHER, on the other hand, is also somewhat analagous to the Web, for it consists of a network of servers which integrally tie into one another. These systems, and the information on them, are quickly being replaced by or put on the Web. Therefore, we shall not explore them in this book.

WHAT SOFTWARE/HARDWARE DO I NEED TO GET ON THE INTERNET?

What's listed below is what you *minimally* need if you want to access the Internet and have a somewhat enjoyable visit. Note that the more you upgrade from this minimum, the more you will enjoy using the Internet. Here's what you need:

- A "486" / 75 megahertz (MH) or larger computer chip with at least 16 megabyte ram of memory.

- A 14,400 bits-per-second (bps) modem.

AND EITHER:

- A Web browser — software which allows you to view documents on the Internet

AND

- An Internet service provider (ISP)

OR

- An on-line service company (America Online, Compuserve, Prodigy, etc.)

If you are a novice don't let all of this terminology scare you. If you are in the process of buying a computer let me assure you that all new computers are Internet capable out of the box. If you already have access to a computer and are having trouble logging on to the Internet, ask someone to help you. Or if you're "surfing," (an Internet term for going from one Web page to another) and your computer seems to be too slow for you, then consult with your local computer store for upgrade options and costs.

On-line Service Companies vs. Internet Service Providers

The pros and cons of using an on-line service over a direct ISP vary. On-line services come with additional services only accessible if you are on their service. The Reproductive & Infertility folders on America Online, which we will discuss in Chapter 5, are such an example. However, you will find that sometimes the Internet runs slower while using these services because of the heavy load of people who subscribe to them.

An Internet service provider can give you some of the extra speed you desire. Their software, however, usually doesn't have any of the pretty graphics and is usually harder to first install. But most ISPs now provide a Web browser and e-mail software with their service, although this may be at an additional cost.

For a novice, however, an on-line service company may be the best way to first get your feet wet on the Internet. Some on-line service companies include America Online, Prodigy, or Compuserve. These companies provide you with user-friendly software which comes on one disk and is all you need to log on to their system and take advantage of the Internet. They *are* the Internet Service Provider. Their software *includes* a Web browser, e-mail, access to newsgroups, and often other services which you will not get with just using an Internet Service Provider alone. Dialing into their system is also easy to do and this dial-up function is an inherent part of their software. But, as previously mentioned, you will sacrifice a certain amount of speed if you choose to access the Internet with an on-line service company.

In order to compete with the on-line service companies, an ISP will usually provide you with a similar service, the software — a dial-up program, Web browser, a newsgroup reader, and e-mail — viewer come as different software programs. Therefore, these programs must be accessed separately when using them on your computer. Some Service Providers still do not supply the e-mail, Web browser or newsgroup reader software, so be sure to ask if they do when you are shopping for a provider. If your ISP supplies an e-mail software, then they will assign you an e-mail address. Once all of the software is loaded you may then log on to their system by using the dial-up software. Once you are successfully logged on then you must open the Web browser software. A home page (usually the Internet Service Provider's or the Web Browser's company) will appear. If you live in a rural community and can't get access to an ISP, an on-line service company may be your only option.

Web Browsers

There are several Web browsers currently available — Netscape Navigator and Microsoft Explorer are two of the more popular ones. On-line services such as America Online, Prodigy, or Compuserve may either have their own Web browsers built into their software or they may employ another commercially available browser application.

In all Web browsers you will notice several icon keys at the top of the page. Let's review a few of these to make your life a little easier.

Back (<) key   Allows you to visit the pages where you previously have been

Forward (>) key   If you went back to find previous pages, "forward" takes you back to where you were beforehand

Stop (X)   Allows you to abandon the current command, useful if it is taking too long to pull up a particular Web site or you decide you no longer want to go to that address.

Newgroups   Allows quick access to looking at newsgroups

Search   Allows quick access to a default search engine(s)

Now — to find a particular Web page or "site" (as it is also commonly referred as) you must type in the Uniform Resource Locator (URL) address in the long window at the top of the page. (Sometimes this is located after the word "Location" or "Address.") Most Web browsers no longer require you to type the *http://* part of the address. The browser understands that it is a Web page you are looking for and automatically processes the information this way. Believe it or not, there is a method to the mayhem of what a URL address means. Let's take a closer look at this, because it will help us in the future by allowing us to locate the source or parent Web pages of the page we are viewing.

Take, for example, the first Web site which is reviewed in Chapter 3. The address of this site is: http://www.vais.net/~travis/firl.html. Let's quickly dissect this site name.

http://
This tells the Web browser that it is a hypertext document that resides on the Web. Some Web browsers no longer need this prefix in a site address and just assume that the address is a Web document and it automatically defaults to this protocol.

www.vais.net/
This is the main or parent Web page — in this case, an Internet Service Provider which provides the computer system where these Web pages physically reside. Note that this address will usually end in either .net, .com, .gov., .org., or .edu suffixes — which, respectively, stand for an Internet service provider, a company, a governmental entity, an organization (usually nonprofit) or an educational institution (usually university or college).

~travis/
This indicates that this is a personal (noted by the tilde) Web page. By typing just the URL address up to this point you will notice that this leads to a gentleman named Travis Low, who has a personal Web page of his own. On this page you can then access the Web page which is featured in this book — The Fertility Information Resource List

firl.html
This is that Web page — With this extention, it is the actual page location of The Fertility Information Resource List. Note the file extension is .html, which also is just .htm in some documents.

Realize that sometimes pages are layered on top of one another and so you may have to erase several of the files/directories until you find the originator — this is true in some very long addresses.

If you type in an address and you get an error message, don't despair — you may have simply typed in the address wrong. A couple items should be noted that may help alleviate problems when typing and entering site addresses. First, don't forget that little squiggly thing (~) if it is in an address. (I was only recently informed by my editor, who is an English major, that the proper term for it is a tilde — pronounced tilda. It is usually found at the upper-left hand corner of your keyboard. The tilde basically just shows that this is a personal (instead of a commercial) Web site.) Anyway, don't forget to put it in an address when it's required, otherwise the browser will not be able to locate the site.

Secondly, when typing in an address for the first time — make sure that you type and enter it exactly. If there are capital letters in the address, make sure that you type in capital letters, or vice-versa. Addresses such as this are known to be *case sensitive* and, once again, a Web browser may not be able to locate the address if it is not typed in properly.

As we will later discuss, one of the main reasons you need to use learn how to use search engines is to locate a site whose address has changed. If you are confident that you have typed in the address correctly, and are still getting an error message that the address could not be located, then it may have "moved," and you need to search for the new address. See Chapter 14 on Learning to Search Properly.

WHAT IF I DON'T HAVE A COMPUTER OF MY OWN?

Anymore, not having your own computer is no longer an excuse for not getting on the Internet. Probably the easiest and least costly way of acquiring access to the Net is "borrowing" time on someone else's computer. Maybe you have a good friend who not only would let you use their computer, but may be able to show you a short-cut or two. Or maybe your employer has the necessary hardware. Mind you, I am not advocating use of your work computer during normal business hours, but normally companies won't mind use of their systems before or after hours (or during lunch if it is available). However, I highly recommend asking permission to use the machines and software if they have not been assigned to you. You probably don't want to tell the boss exactly what you're looking at, for privacy's sake, but you may want to just inform your boss that you're in search of some "hard to find" info which is personal in nature.

One avenue you don't want to overlook is your local library. More and more libraries are providing terminals to access the Internet — most of them, of course, have free access! (Although some limit the hours of use.) And, as usual, librarians will eagerly to help you get acclimated to using the machines. Some libraries are even now offering classes on how to use the Internet.

Another good public place is your nearby school. Your hard-earned tax dollars or tuition, if its a private school, should gain you access to computers available there.

In some of the larger cities it is becoming more and more popular to combine Internet access with eateries or coffee shops. Patrons may then pay an hourly rate and enjoy surfing with a cappucino or a light bit to eat. Check your local Yellow Pages to see if any of these shops are available in your area.

Finally, if you want to spend a bit of money, check with your local electronics store for the newest gadget which will allow you Internet access through your television! The systems are more expensive than the above option, but are much cheaper than buying your own computer system. Some can be purchased as low as $500 with a $20/month service charge for Internet access.

HOW TO USE THIS BOOK

This book primarily consists of reviews of neatly categorized Web pages under respective headings. You will find the URL address listed for each one under its title. I have purposely underlined all links (just like they appear on the appropriate Web page at time of publication of this book) to other sites and subpages in the reviews of the Web pages. I did this to make your searching for a particular bit of information a little easier.

Although Web sites are some of the best and easiest resources for information, do not overlook the support aspect that mailing lists, bulletin boards, newsgroups, and chat rooms provide (discussed in Chapter 5). Finally, since the Internet is an ever-expanding informational source, we will explore ways of searching for specific information you may want or to find other new sites which pop up on the Internet continuously in Chapter 14.

One final tip when using this book: most Web browsers contain a place to bookmark or list favorite Web sites, which can then be quickly pulled up in future viewings by simply clicking on that icon. Find this function on your browser and use it. It will make revisiting your favorite sites so much easier — since you will not have to retype or remember addresses once these are entered as bookmarks.

This quick overview should have you set. So let's go surfing and explore some of the wonderful resources the Internet has to offer!

CHAPTER 2

PROFESSIONAL FERTILITY WEB SITES

To get you started, I've organized the first couple of chapters in this book with Web sites which cover the whole realm of infertility. This first chapter of Web reviews features sites which are owned and operated by formal organizations (many non-profit groups) which interact with doctors or other medical personnel on a continuous basis. Because of this interaction they are very reliable sources of information. The information itself on the pages tends to get updated very frequently also, so that you have the latest and greatest information at your fingertips. In the next chapter, some personal Web pages — those created and maintained by only one person who has probably experience infertility firsthand — are reviewed. Although these may not be updated as frequently, the personal flair they provide is worth the trip. In either case, all of the sites in these first two chapters will be a good "starting place" to begin your investigation of infertility information on the Internet and I highly suggest bookmarking all of them in your browser for quick future reference. By doing this you may then easily access other sites that we will discuss in this book. There is information "a plenty" here — happy surfing!

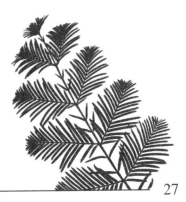

InterNational Council on Infertility Information Dissemination

(http://www.inciid.org)

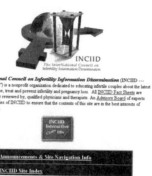

The InterNational Council on Infertility Information Dissemination (INCIID --- pronounced "inside") is a nonprofit organization dedicated to educating infertile couples about the latest methods to diagnose, treat and prevent infertility and pregnancy loss. All INCIID Fact Sheets are either written by, or reviewed by, qualified physicians and therapists. An Advisory Board of experts oversees the activities of INCIID to ensure that the contents of this site are in the best interests of medical consumers.

One of the largest, oldest, and best formatted on-line organizations providing infertility information is the InterNational Council on Infertility Information Dissemination. Commonly known as INCIID (pronounced "inside") this non-profit organization has an extensive mission — to provide *accurate* on-line information to those experiencing infertility. That is why it must be listed here at the start of this book, since this site entails so much unique and sound medical information regarding infertility. I cannot over-emphasize that a trip to this site is a MUST for all infertility patients.

The INCIID Backgrounder (provided under the About INCIID link) is quite a provoking tale of the development of this Web site and the organization. Some may call it coincidence, some might call it fate — only you can decide why things happened the way they did for the founders of this organization and site. That's all I'll say — *you'll* have to pull up the page to find out the rest.

The INCIID Site Index opens to many wonderful sources of information. Be sure not to miss their Index of Fact Sheets and Auditorium Transcripts. Under this link you will find an extensive Glossary of Infertility Terms and reproduction techniques. Basic Infertility Testing is a "must read" for everyone. It lays out all of the typical tests involved in a *good* extensive infertility workup, including all of the blood tests which should be run for hormones. It even details the specifics of these tests as to corresponding days on which each should be pulled and the "normal" levels into which they should fall. Some of the other great informational fact sheets available under this link include:

- Pregnancy hCG Beta Chart

- Recommended Clinics Requirements for ART Procedures

- ICSI Offers New Hope for Couples with Severe Male Factor

- Immunology May Be Key to Recurrent Pregnancy Loss

- Reproductive Immunology Bibliography

- Insurance Coverage for Infertility Treatment

- Specialized Ultrasound Screening Can Be Key to Predicting Implantation Odds

Recently they have just added an extensive list of Bulletin Board & Chats where advice is given and moderated by members of their professional advisory board.

There is so much more to this site that it's hard to put within the confines of these few pages. Much, much more information continues to be added as technology and need evolve. Once you have a chance to visit this site, you will see for yourself how it alone may become your one stop shop for infertility information.

Fertilitext

(http://www.fertilitext.org)

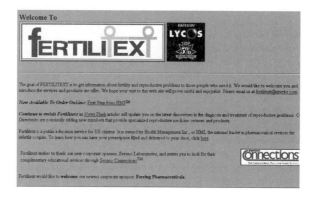

Fertilitext was founded in 1995 with its mission to "provide educational information and referrals to individuals who want to conceive or may be experiencing infertility." It was one of the original sites solely dedicated to providing information on fertility.

This site provides basic, quick, easily readable information. The information laid out on this site is primarily directed toward those just starting to educate themselves about their fertility, thus, it's a great place to get your feet wet if want to find out:

How Do I Know When I Am Most Fertile?

How Common is Infertility?

When Do I Need to Seek Help from a Physician?

How Can I Know which Doctors are Specialists?

What's involved in an Infertility Evaluation?

What do all those Medical Terms Mean?

What are the Most Common Causes of Infertility?

What are the Most Common Treatments of Infertility?

Also included on this Web site are pages discussing Information on Prescription Drugs and Insurance / Managed Care Verification of Benefits and Reimbursement. The fertility drug information is good, and easily readable. The article on insurance is a bit subjective, but it is linked to an excellent resource — a Sample Letter which you can use to send to your insurance company to verify upcoming coverage of a infertility treatment.

There is also a referral section of their page to physicians, sperm banks, egg donors, pharmacy distributors, and other support groups. However, please be aware that this list is also by no means inclusive and that, unlike RESOLVE (discussed in Chapter 4), these participants must pay a fee to be listed in this directory.

One excellent resource that no one will want to miss on this site is the Help on Specific Questions service which Fertilitext provides. When I came across this my eyes about popped out of my head. Here is a FREE service where you can ask a *trained medical staff* about any questions you may have regarding your fertility, treatments, etc. As you can image — their e-mail is flooded most of the time, and it they say may take up to a couple weeks to get a reply — but, hcy, it's free! (Similarly discussed in Chapter 6, is Mediconsult.com, another excellent free medical consultation service.)

As with many other fertility organizations and companies which have Web sites, Fertilitext also offers books, tapes, and CDs on fertility-related issues which can be purchased. Check it out!

Infertility Resources

(http://www.ihr.com/infertility/)

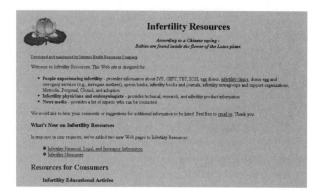

Infertility Resources was created and is maintained by Dr. Clifford Bernstein who has worked many years not only in the mental health field but also as a computer systems analyst. He has put this unique blend of experience to work when he started his company Internet Health Resources (IHR) in 1994.

IHR's mission is twofold: to provide the extensive Infertility Resources Web site (listed above), and to provide marketing opportunities for infertility organizations (listed on IHR's homepage - http://www.ihr.com/ihrhome.html). With regards to the latter mission, this Web site links visitors to a large array of Web pages which contain specific Fertility Clinics who have chosen to "advertise" through the use of Dr. Bernstein's page. You will be surprised at *how many* clinics are on the Web now. Many of these clinics also do provide infertility resources, but to minimize the length of this book I have chosen not to highlight all of the individual ones (except only one that I MUST in Chapter 6.) But if you cannot find one that may interest you through this site, then check out either Appendix B which lists all the current ones I could find or Chapter 14 on Learning How to Search Properly to help you locate nearby clinics which may have their own presence on the Web.

Because of IHR's mission, the Infertility Resources page is extremely well organized, and numerous links are associated with each of the outlined topics. A "must read" on this Web site is Infertility Treatment. This page opens to a vast array of other links which include everything from getting started, to specifics on ART, to surrogacy and even new information on Choosing the Sex of Your Child.

On the Additional Educational Articles page make sure not to miss The Visible Embryo. WOW!! — was my first impression. This shows the first four weeks of conception and has capabilities to blow your mind away if you have multimedia capabilities on your computer. Also on this page is something I'm sure we all can relate to — Handling Conflicts Between Work & Infertility Care. I haven't seen much written on this topic so here's reason in itself to get on that computer and on the Web! Also listed under this page is Women's Health Web Sites, some even searchable.

As a final note, in addition to the vast links listed under Fertility Clinics, you'll also find direct links to:

- Donor Egg and Surrogacy Services
- Natural Methods — (an alternative approach, if nothing else it helps you deal with the stress of infertility)
- Online Pharmacies Selling Infertility Medication (some at decent prices)
- Infertility Books, Articles, Newsletters, and Videotapes
- Infertility Newsgroups and List Discussion (good, quick, easily accessible reference — more information on these are covered in detail in Chapter 5)
- Infertility Organizations — most listed in this book
- Adoption Resources — I list many of these in Chapter 10, but I now realize an entire book can be written on these resources alone — (*maybe next book*)

And the Web being the ever evolving creature it is, many more topics will follow, I'm sure.

Home Arts : Infertility Update

(http://homearts.com/depts/health/37upf1.htm)

Home Arts is a commercial Web site dedicated to the lifestyle of women. Owned by the Hearst Corporation, a leading communications company, Home Arts provides a forum for women to meet and share information on everything from cooking to love to health. Under their Body & Soul link you will find this page on their *Infertility Update*. This site includes information on Where to Start, as well as Treatment News for Men and Women. Several other articles include The Cost of Conceiving and a review of fertility clinics under The Business of Babies. Before you leave this site Join the Conversation About Infertility on their online bulletin board.

Ferre Institute

(http://members.aol.com/ferreinf/ferre.html)

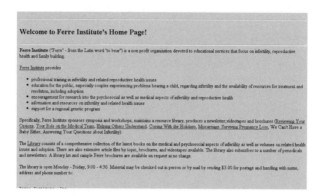

Don't like the idea of spending that much money on books? Then you must visit the Ferre Institute site. Begun in 1978, Ferre Institute is a nonprofit organization whose main mission is to provide infertility information. Their site is very basic but provides inexpensive access to its <u>Library</u> which contains a huge selection of books, journals, pamphlets, videotapes, and cassettes. Located in Utica, NY, the material may be checked out in person, or you may receive material through the mail for $3.00 to handle shipping and handling. Their address, phone number, fax and e-mail address is located on their home page. A few of their pamphlets are located on-line and include:

<u>Reviewing Your Options</u>

<u>Your Role on the Medical Team</u>

<u>Helping Others Understand</u>

<u>Coping with the Holidays</u>

<u>Miscarriage: Surviving Pregnancy Loss</u>

New York Online Access to Health

(http://www.noah.cuny.edu/pregnancy/fertility.html)

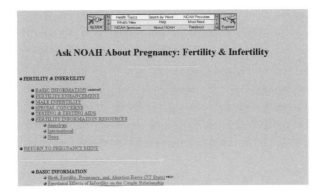

The New York Online Access to Health (otherwise known as NOAH™) was originally founded by a partnership between the City University of New York, the New York Academy of Medicine, New York Metropolitan Reference and Research Library Agency, and the New York Public Library. Started over 25 years ago, NOAH™ has grown with the help of other sponsors such as the March of Dimes, U.S. Healthcare, the New York University Medical Center and Queens Borough Public Library. NOAH™ has for its mission to "provide high quality full-text health information for consumers that is accurate, timely, relevant and unbiased." The organization began their online venture in 1995.

This particular address links you to their site on *Fertility and Infertility*. Although the site contains little original information, dozens of links have been diligently found and catagorized into topics such as <u>Basic Information</u>, <u>Fertility Enhancement</u>, <u>Male Infertility</u>, <u>Special Concerns</u>, <u>Testing and Testing Aids</u>, and other <u>Fertility Information Resources</u>.

Child of My Dreams Resource Center_{sm}

(http://www.child-dream.com)

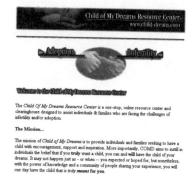

The *Child Of My Dreams Resource Center* is a one-stop, online resource center and clearinghouse designed to assist individuals & families who are facing the challenges of infertility and/or adoption.

The Mission...

The mission of *Child of My Dreams* is to provide individuals and families seeking to have a child with encouragement, support and inspiration. More importantly, COMD aims to instill in individuals the belief that if you **truly** want a child, you can and **will** have the child of your dreams. It may not happen just as - or when -- you expected or hoped for, but nonetheless, with the power of knowledge and a community of people sharing your experience, you will one day have the child that is truly *meant* for you.

A last minute entry into this book was the Child of My Dreams Resource Center^{SM}, which I had to place in this first chapter of Web sites This site was not even officially on-line when this book went to the printer, but I was fortunate enough to be given a "sneak preview" of the site — and from the looks of it, it's one you'll definitely want to visit!

"Born" from an idea between its two cofounders, Cindy Simons Bennett (who adopted after a bout with cancer) and Francesca Linquist (founder of the HOPE Web site — see Chapter 4) created this site, and it's like no other in this book. Child of My Dreams strives to be a "one-stop online resource center" focused on both infertility *and* adoption resources. The mission of Child of My Dreams is to provide individuals and families seeking to have a child with encouragement, support and inspiration.

Some of the *unique* features which the site will have include:

➡ A constantly updated searchable database of national and international infertility clinics and adoption agencies;

➡ Information on how to choose an infertility clinic or adoption agency, including a listing of appropriate fees, questions to ask, key services to seek, and a "good clinic" checklist;

➡ Listings of organizations and institutions that provide loans for infertility and adoption procedures;

➡ Member-created content and areas where members can share helpful hints, journals, poetry, online graffiti and photographs; and

➡ Online baby showers and other personal celebrations

In addition to these features, the site will also offer online forums hosted with professionals in the field, bulletin boards, chat sessions, and many other goodies. My gut feeling is that it will become one of the prestigious fertility/adoption sites on the Web.

CHAPTER 3
PERSONAL FERTILITY WEB SITES

Although formal organizations may be able to provide the most accurate and comprehensive fertility information, there's nothing like a good Web site personally designed by someone who has their own twist on the subject. Information on these Web sites may be based on personal experience and/or their own opinion. As always, be a wise consumer on the Internet and always cross check information with other sources and your own physician!

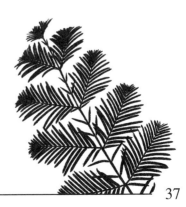

Fertility Information Resource List

There's a tilde in this one — don't forget it!

(http://www.vais.net/~travis/firl.html)

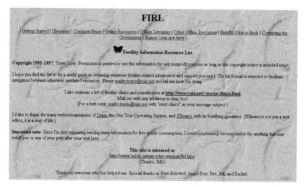

Let me start by saying that, I'll admit — this site is not the fanciest and does not include all the illustrious bells and whistles which could be used on a Web page (although in time I imagine this aspiring computer wiz will add these features.) But, as a fellow engineer, I recognize that content is what really matters — and this might be the "Mother of all Infertility Information Web sites." This personal site is basically an excellent collection of well laid out hyperlinks to other Web pages, e-mail addresses, newsgroup listings, and other related infertility information. As previously mentioned, the site was created by Travis Low — a software engineer who, as you can imagine, has been personally touched by the bite of infertility in his own life.

Travis has done an exceptional job at organizing this site and has put together a <u>Getting Started</u> section which includes hot buttons to related sites which will aid anyone who is starting to battle infertility, as well as items that may have been overlooked by us veterans. He has also added his two cents worth of advice in his <u>Common Sense</u> section on taking charge of your situation — a *must read!*

Pineland Press' Fertility Information Table of Contents

(http://www.pinelandpress.com/toc.html)

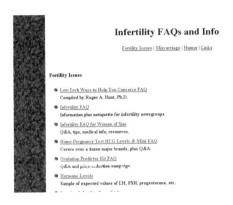

This site is an excellent resource for it provides information I have not seen elsewhere. As a first stop at this site I highly recommend looking at <u>Low-Tech Ways to Help You Conceive</u> by Roger A. Hunt, Ph.D. The information on this link is closely based on information in the book *Taking Charge of Your Fertility* by Toni Wenchler. This site and/or book is "Fertility 101" and should be a must read for anyone who wants to attain *or* avoid pregnancy — for it shows you how to identify *all* your fertility signs — more than just looking at your basal body temperature (BBT). (After battling infertility as long as I have, I thought I knew everything there was to know about my body — until I recently read this book. However, be warned that it, too, is not all-inclusive and should only be used as a piece of the puzzle.) Needless to say, the information in this one page *alone* is worth a trip to this site. You need not even buy the book — most of the useful information in it is contained in this web site. There even is a search function in the site which you can use to identify related problems. And don't miss out on the fertility chart which you can download into EXCEL spreadsheets.

In addition to this most valuable basic information there are also some other unique topics including:

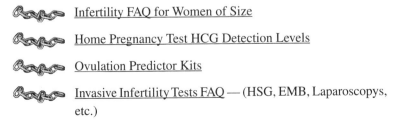

Infertility FAQ for Women of Size

Home Pregnancy Test HCG Detection Levels

Ovulation Predictor Kits

Invasive Infertility Tests FAQ — (HSG, EMB, Laparoscopys, etc.)

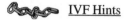 IVF Hints

Discount Fertility Medication (How & Where to Get It)

Recurrent Pregnancy Loss Testing

This site also has an excellent link to one of the broadest Miscarriage Support and Information Resource lists I've seen.

One of the more lighthearted bits on this page is the Infertility Sniglets in the "Humor Section." If you're having a bad day and the hormones have got you or your spouse in an uproar, roar back in laughter with a look into this link. Only couples in our shoes would truly appreciated its humor! By the way — regarding the other items in this "Humor Section" — don't ask me! I'll let *you* find out the underlying story behind those photos from Roger himself.

Waiting For Stork: Infertility Resources

(http://www.cyberspacepr.com/infertility.html)

Waiting For Stork is a wonderfully written Web site brought to you by Cyberspace PR. In answer to the question Are We Infertile, this site helps you deal with infertility by laying out some sage advise in their sections on Finding the Right Doctor, Finding a Support Group, Welcome to High-Tech Infertility Treatment: It's a ride on a runaway train, and Grief and Infertility: Handling Miscarriage or the Death of Your Dreams. This wonderful resource also contains some gems like:

How Does Infertility Affect Our Friends

A Christian and a Jewish Rabbi Share Their Thoughts on Infertility

The Emotional Aspects of Infertility, and

A Prayer For My Wife on Mother's Day.

Debbie's Infertility Information Pages

(http://www.applink.net/~akima/wishing.htm)

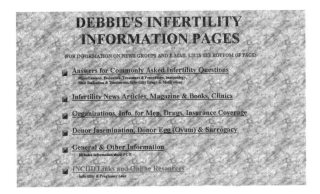

This is just one of the many Web pages that computer wiz Debbie Shavel has constructed. (Check out her index of other Web pages on http://applink.net/~akima.)

Like Travis Low's page, it is a great compilation of infertility hyperlinks to other sites on the Internet. For those of you with computer speakers, she has also added sound for your listening enjoyment while surfing through her pages. In addition to the Answers for Commonly Asked Infertility Questions, be sure not to miss the link to Infertility News Articles, Magazines & Books, Clinics. She has done an excellent job combing the Web to find many articles in popular magazines which have had feature articles on infertility.

D.A.M.'s Infertility Resources

(http://www.geocities.com/TheTropics/Shores/2713/infertility.html)

As you might come to realize with time, many personal Web sites reviewed in this book will be extentions of the URL address "www.geocities.com." That is because Geocities is an online provider of free personal Web site space. They make money by providing a network of Web page creation products and by advertising on their well trafficked site.

D.A.M's (David and Mel's) Infertility Resources is such a site. Although Mel suffers from PCO (see Chapter 7), much of the resources on the site are devoted to links to overall infertility and adoption. They also have a unique situation in that they both are in the military, which brings with it some other challenges for this couple on top of their infertility.

Infertility..... by Kansas

(http://www.geocities.com/Heartland/Meadows/4160/fertility.html)

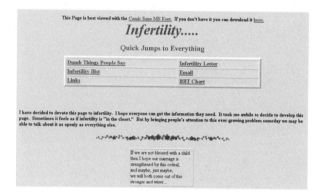

This site created by Kansas Allen offers a couple of my personal favorite tidbits. Be sure to check out <u>Dumb Things People Say</u> to a couple experiencing fertility problems. I believe you will relate and will definitely get a good chuckle from reading through these timeless ignorant comments people often make to those of us going through this ordeal. Another one of my favorites is a link she found on the topic of <u>Marriage: In Sickness and in Health...and Infertility?</u> This article wisely lays out how each of the sexes deals with the infertility crisis and what you can do to keep the love alive through such a trying time.

CHAPTER 4
EMOTIONAL/FINANCIAL SUPPORT WEB SITES

Childless Mother
by
Louise C. Taylor

I am a childless mother.
There is an empty hole in my heart
Where my child is supposed to be.
Where there should be squeals and laughter
There is nothing but mind-numbing silence.
And look, there, in the corner sitting idly,
Waiting, is a child's rocker, my rocker—
The rocker that I used to sit in and imagine
Rocking my baby instead of just a doll.
And I realize, that as empty as that rocker seems,
My arms feel even heavier with the emptiness.
How can emptiness feel so heavy?
That emptiness carries my broken dreams,
My disappointments, my resentment.
Flutterby kisses never shared,
Laughter never heard,
Tears never brushed away
All weigh more than a child ever will.
There is an empty hole in my heart
Where my child is supposed to be.
I am a childless mother.

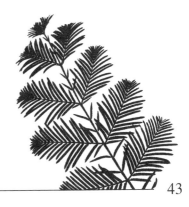

More than anything, conserving the resources that you have is imperative when you are going through the infertility experience. The two resources which seem to get used more than others are your emotional and financial ones. As I mentioned in the introduction of this book one of the key ways to get through this battle alive is to get support — both financially and emotionally.

Many couples I've known have literally mortgaged their homes or "maxed out" all of their credit cards to try "one last IVF attempt." Even if the attempt worked, the couple is faced with years of additional debt. As many of us battling this can attest, the main reason couples are tempted to do this is because most of the advanced reproductive techniques (IVF, GIFT) are not covered by insurance in most states. More and more couples are becoming politically active in order to push change in this area. I have included a couple Web sites in this chapter which particularly focus on financial aid and ways of getting the most out of your insurance — make sure not to miss these.

RESOLVE

(http://www.resolve.org)

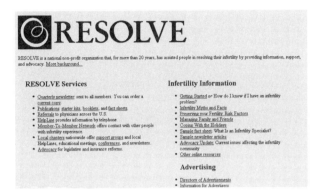

Most couples battling infertility have at least heard of RESOLVE — our nation's first and largest infertility support organization. If you have not checked them out, or if you keep putting off going to that first meeting — then be sure to check out what you're missing on their national web site!

Although there is a nominal charge, RESOLVE's facts sheets are second to none as far as concise technical information. The list of subjects covered spans the entire realm of the infertility nightmare: from treatment and coping to alternative medicines or surgery to child-free living or adoption.

RESOLVE's newsletters are also superb. Some sample newsletters and facts sheets are available on their Web site. Many other fact sheets are available to non-members for purchase, but are substaintually discounted with membership. However, the quarterly newsletter can only be obtained through membership (currently $45/year — and well worth it).

Some of the sample fact sheets listed on their site include:

- Infertility Myths & Facts

- What is an Infertility Specialist?

- Coping with the Holidays

- Managing Family & Friends (one of my favorites — learn great comeback lines to educate the fertile world!)

In addition to the concise information and support which RESOLVE offers, the organization continues to supply needed advocacy to our legislative bodies, in order to push for reform which will aid infertile persons nationwide.

HOPE : Infertility Support

(http:// members.aol.com/FrancescaQ/HOPE.html)

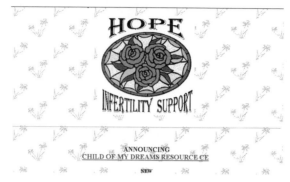

So appropriately named, one of my personal favorites, is the HOPE Web site. In conjunction with the HOPE folders on America Online's Personal Empowerment Network, this site was designed in 1995 and is maintained by Francesca "Franki" Linquist. Being a volunteer support forum host for AOL, she came up with the idea for the HOPE folders out of her own need to find others who were also battling infertility and understood. As the support groups grew on the HOPE folders (see Chapter 5 on how to access bulletin boards) this Web page followed to provide a collection of information discussed on the HOPE boards.

To me it gives such true emotional support which is so desperately needed in the trying times associated with infertility. Upon visiting this site, one can't help but automatically "feel" like a part of this family. Membership into HOPE requires only participation and an understanding of the infertility experience.

As a part of the Web page, the owner of the site tells her own story, which, in itself, can't help but to inspire all who read it. The site also includes the HOPE Family Album — a compilation of other individual HOPE members, their own inspirational stories, HOPE member birthdays, inspirational news, stories, and some technical information.

The HOPE web site includes many other features such as:

- A Chat Schedule on AOL for Hope Members
- Alphabet Soup — A Compilation of acronyms used on the boards and throughout the web site
- Hope's Happy Thoughts — Motivational & Inspirational Poetry
- Alternative Treatments
- Recommended Books on Infertility
- How to Choose an RE — a "must read" with great questions to ask when your interviewing prospective doctors

Many other topics are listed, and more web pages are "in the works."

ONNA

(http://www.thought-crimes.com/onna/)

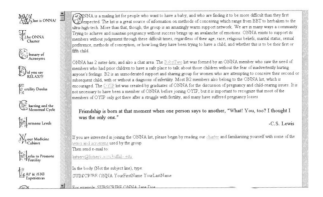

Very similar to the concept of HOPE, there is ONNA — a web page created after a mailing list dealing with infertility and chats on the Internet Relay Chat (IRC) system had been taking place between a group fighting infertility for sometime. ONNA's homepage, however, is a "don't miss site", for it not only provides support but also supplies extremely useful information and tools. Much of the information available on this site is a cooperative effort of the members of ONNA and include:

- BBT Charts which can be downloaded into EXCEL spreadsheets

- Explanations of the Typical Menstrual Cycle

- Information on Ovulation Predictor Kits

- Comparison of Home Pregnancy Tests

- "Low-Tech" Home Medical Treatments

- Herbal Treatments to Aid Fertility (one of the best I've seen on the Net)

For this reason, I'd advise anyone "starting out" on the journey to visit this site. Or for older veterans, its a good resource to re-evaluate if you feel you've already tried everything.

Using a hot button on their home page, you can also subscribe easily to their any of their mailing lists. In addition to the ONNA list, there also is a mailing list for those trying for their second child and experiencing difficulties — Baby Two.

For "graduates" of ONNA, there is the OYIP (Oh Yeah/Yippee I'm Pregnant) mailing list and Web page all of which can be easily accessed through this site. To participate in their on-line chats, use of the IRC system is thoroughly explained on their site, as well. Access to the system can be simply obtained by downloading some files.

Did I forget to mention what ONNA means? Oh well, I guess I'll have to let *you* find that out. An "acronyms" listing of what it means, as well as other commonly used terminology used on ONNA's mailing list and Web pages, is also available on their Home page.

Infertility Helper Magazine

(http://www.helping.com/family/iy/ih.html)

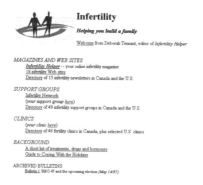

Infertility Helper claims to be "your online infertility support magazine." Started in 1995 by Robin Hilborn, this quarterly Canadian magazine is filled with great articles on fertility enhancement. Some recent issues include <u>What do I tell them at work?</u> — an article dealing with how to juggle career and treatment. Another article, <u>Ethics of the new reproductive technologies,</u> consists of a five panel discussion on the topic. And, for a bit of humor (although, sad to say, is the truth) check out the article in the September '96 edition entitled <u>A view from the broom closet,</u> which is a man's perspective of the steps required to "getting tested." For a $25 subscription, you may also get the Magazine in hard form by writing the Infertility Helper at 36 Norwood Road, Toronto, Ontario, M4E 2S2 Canada.

Hannah's Prayer

(http://www.hannah.org)

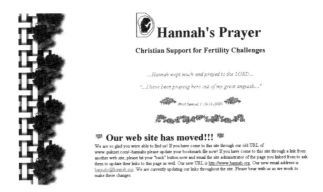

Do you often wonder "why God is letting this happen to you"? Or are you having some ethical problems regarding upcoming infertility treatment decisions? Then check out Hannah's Prayer. Rick and Jenni Saake, a couple from California, created this Web site as an alternative to those who wanted more of a Christian viewpoint on the whole frustrating situation. Not only does this site cover infertility, but it also extends support to those who have experienced stillbirth and early infant death.

This site offer many resources not found easily elsewhere and include:

- Pregnancy Loss & Early Infant Death Resources

- High Risk Pregnancy Resources (Bed Rest, Multiples, Subsequent Pregnancy after loss)

- General Grief Resources

- Christian Based Ethical/Moral Views on Fertility Related Issues

- Thoughts & Stories of Inspiration

In addition, Hannah's Prayer publishes a quarterly newsletter — Hannah-to-Hannah. Hannah's Prayer also has a live chat room via IRC, and downloadable software to use IRC is available on this site as well.

Writings of Infertile Couples

(http://www.teleport.com/~lsundae/infert.htm)

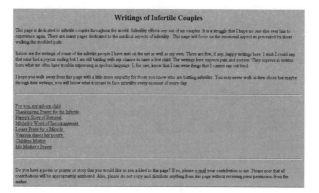

It seems very appropriate that this page is simplistic in nature. Being a gifted poet herself, Louise Taylor, the owner of this page, began writing about her own infertility and now has started collecting others' writings about their losses. As I have previously mentioned, sometimes writing about your own difficult experiences can be extremely therapeutic, and this site is an example of that. Hopefully you will find solace in reading through some of the poems and writings on this site. Maybe you will even have one to add yourself. Some of my personal favorites from her collection include a <u>Thanksgiving Prayer for the Infertile</u> as well as her <u>Childless Mother</u> poem featured at the beginning of this chapter.

Fertile Thoughts (Formally Infertility Penpals)

(http://www.bluestars.com/clinic/index.shtml)

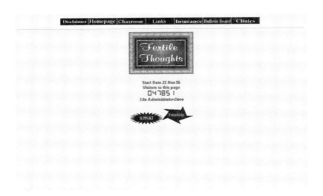

Getting fed up with the fact that your insurance doesn't cover infertility treatments? Then you MUST check out this Web site! Fertile Thoughts was created by a couple in Mississippi who have battled infertility for 8 years and are fighting back by offering this informative and interactive web site. This site offers invaluable information such as:

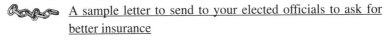 A sample letter to send to your elected officials to ask for better insurance

State Infertility Laws

Getting the most out of your insurance

How to get an Adoption Loan without Collateral

World Infertility Clinics with Maps

Infertility Drug Information

And, while you're visiting their site, why not browse the pen pal section to find a friend who is also in your shoes to share experiences, ask advice, or just vent? Open and private chat rooms are also available for real time discussions.

CHAPTER 5
INFERTILITY MAILING LISTS, NEWSGROUPS, BULLETIN BOARDS, and CHAT ROOMS

I always feel very sad when I hear of a parent whose child has died. I sometimes believe that I know what that pain feels like. I grieve every month for the hope/dream of a child that doesn't come. I never had the opportunity to hold my child, or kiss him/her, or even name my child. I don't know what my child would have looked like, but I still feel as though I am a grieving parent.

I am tired of pretending to be happy when I hear of someone's pregnancy.

I am tired of pretending that sex is anything more than a means to an end.

I am tired of pretending that I'm not bitter.

Why me?

Julie (Day 2)— posting from AOL's HOPE: Infertility Support folder

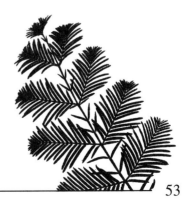

Probably the best thing about these features on the Internet is the personal one-on-one support which they can give. Although each of these posting mechanisms are a bit different from one another, newsgroups, bulletin boards and mailing lists provide a great support vehicle — mainly because of their interactive capabilities, which a Web site rarely offers. As e-mail and the Internet has come of age, many people combating infertility figured out early that this was both an excellent mechanism to share information in a confidential atmosphere and a vehicle to express their emotions to other people who could relate to the sincere hurt that they were feeling.

However, a word of warning before we get into explaining the specifics of each. I have seen some real emotions come across these types of media — so beware. You *may* get your own feelings hurt (ironically, since the main purpose of these groups is to provide *support*) and have some personal convictions occasionally slammed by others. Just remember that people in general say stupid things sometimes because they are so wrapped up in their own troubles — even if the cross they're carrying is the same as yours. For this reason, many of these lists are posting "netiquette" guidelines on the do's and don'ts of how to post. Topics such as religion, politics, etc., tend to become very heated sometimes. After you have had a chance to join or view these lists you will see what I mean, especially if you become active in placing posts.

MAILING LISTS

Accessing each of these sources differs a bit from one another, and each has its own advantages and disadvantages. Mailing lists provide the easiest and probably most accessible posting tool for everyone. To join a mailing list, usually all one must do is to send a standard e-mail message to the list you want to join. Some of the more popular mailing lists follow. The first address should be sent via e-mail to subscribe and unsubscribe to the list. The second address is used to post a message to the group.

THE ILIST

The Infertility Support List (ILIST) is one of the oldest infertility mailing lists. It was created by Toni Bachman who wanted to have a more private forum for support in dealing with infertility. Since that time, the ilist has moved around and is currently at Duke University. The most unique aspect of this list is that you will literally meet people all over the globe who are also in your shoes! At the present time, biographies are kept on members wishing to share their stories, so that other members might be able to hook up with other individuals who have similar diagnosis or are undergoing the same treatments. You can subscribe to the ilist by sending e-mail to:

majordomo@acpub.duke.edu

In the text of your letter simply type "subscribe ilist" (without the quotation marks). To discontinue receiving messages, send e-mail to same address, but type "unsubscribe ilist."

If you have some special requirements about subscribing (such as needing to subscribe under a different address than the one you use to send the subscription message), please send mail with a description of how you would like the ilist administrator to help you with your subscription to:

ilist-owner@acpub.duke.edu

To send a message to the group send e-mail to:

ilist@acpub.duke.edu

ONNA

As previously mentioned in Chapter 4, ONNA started out as a mailing list. It has since grown by addition of the Web page which has a direct link to subscribe to this list. If you do not have Internet access but have only e-mail, you can still subscribe to the list by sending mail to:

listserve@listserv.acsu.buffalo.edu

In the text (not subject) simply type "subscribe onna" (without the quotation marks). To discontinue receiving messages, send e-mail to same address but type "signoff onna."

To send a message to the group send e-mail to:

onna@listserv.acsu.buffalo.edu

LADIES-IN-WAITING

Ladies-in-waiting is a Christian support mailing list that was started by Julie and John Donahue back in 1995. After subscribing to AOL and discovering the advantages of e-mail and the Web, Julie created the list as an alternative for talking with other Christian women who were dealing not only with the other aspects of infertility, but with the ethical and spiritual ones as well. Similar to ONNA, a Web site has recently been formed for this mailing list and is located at:

http://members.aol.com/ladenwaitn/main.htm

This Web page is still in the making and is used as a general forum to help "members" of the mailing list to not only identify other members easily also to find other members with like diagnosis for additional support and information. Unlike other mailing list, however you can only subscribe to this list by visiting their home page (only viewable with frames capability) and filling out their form. You will then be placed on their mailing list.

Some other mailing lists follow below for more specific situations. Each will send you a message back describing how to post a message to the specific group and how to unsubscribe.

DIAGNOSTIC MAILING LISTS

Endometriosis   listserve@listserv.dartmouth.edu

In the text (not subject — leave this blank) type "subscribe witsendo <your last name, first name>" (without the quotation marks).

PCO   pco-request@lists.best.com

In the text (not subject — leave this blank) type only "subscribe" (without the quotation marks).

Fortility (over 40)   fortility-request@columbia.edu

In the text (not subject — leave this blank) type only "subscribe" (without the quotation marks).

ADOPTION MAILING LISTS

Domestic   listserve@sjuvm.stjohns.edu

In the text (not subject — leave this blank) type "subscribe adoption <your last name, first name>" (without the quotation marks).

Russian   listproc@list.serve.com

In the text (not subject — leave this blank) type "a.parent.russ <your last name, first name>" (without the quotation marks).

Cross-Cultural   hctahnee@umich.edu or kja@umich.edu

In the text simply request to join

ALTERNATIVE

Surrogacy   See www.surrogacy.com in Chapter 10

Childfree   majordomo@teleport.com

In the text (not subject — leave this blank) type "subscribe childfree <your mailname@youremailaddress>" (without the quotation marks).

To send a message to the group send e-mail to:

childfree@teleport.com

MISCARRIAGE

Miscarriage after Infertility

listserv@listserv.acsu.bufflo.edu

In the text type "subscribe mai" (without the quotation marks). This list requires a bio/your story which will be approved by the list owner prior to your subscription. (This is done for your extra security and privacy.)

Christian Pregnancy Loss Support

See www.geocities.com/Wellesley/2458 in Chapter 9

PREGNANCY

After Infertility

external-majordomo@palladium.corp.sgi.com

In the text (not subject — leave this blank) simply type "subscribe <your mailname@youremailaddress>" (without the apostrophes).

After Miscarriage

pam-request@fensende.com

In the text (not subject — leave this blank) type only "subscribe" (without the apostrophes).

Subsequent Pregnancy after Loss

SPALS-request@inforamp.net

Leave subject and text blank. This list is for any pregnancy after infertility or other loss.

Unlike a conventional e-mail address, most mailing list subscriptions are handled by a computer, therefore use of them is virtually automatic if you have e-mail. Shortly after you send an e-mail to subscribe to a list you will receive verification that you have been added to the list and you will then start receiving postings from the mailing list from others who have joined.

Besides the ease of joining and using mailing lists, another advantage of using them is that they are somewhat confidential. Unlike bulletin boards and newsgroups where postings reside on an on-line service or even the Internet, you must "join" to view the postings of mailing lists. Some mailing lists will even require that a brief survey be filled out upon joining to weed out "weirdos" (most mailing lists are monitored for protection of their users). For this reason, complete anonymity cannot be maintained on some mailing lists. Probably the single most reason, however, for subscribing to a mailing list is to gain specific information from another individual who may have a similar diagnosis or is undergoing a specific treatment plan. Literally hundreds of people subscribe to and use mailing lists daily, so it's fairly possible to easily find a person who is riding in the same seat of the infertility rollercoaster as you are. The benefits of using a mailing list may best be illustrated by the use of one by a friend of mine. She was lamenting to me on the phone one night that she would love to find a person to talk to who was taking Lupron for endometriosis treatments. I told her about mailing lists and how she could use them to get this information. She then simply subscribed to one of these lists, asked the question, and received many helpful replies.

The main disadvantage of using mailing lists, however, is the problem of a continuously congested mailbox. If you subscribe to some of these mailing lists, be prepared to typically receive over a hundred pieces of mail in a day! Therefore, you will need to be a dedicated reader or you may only want to subscribe to a list when you need a particular question answered or require additional support.

NEWSGROUPS

Similar to mailing lists, newsgroups are discussion forums which use postings for sharing information. There are literally tens of thousands of newgroups on the Internet that cover everything from basket weaving to engineering. However, unlike mailing lists, newsgroups use the concept of postings which are placed on a type of bulletin board on the Internet. Because of this, you must have access to obtaining this information off of the Internet to be able to subscribe, view, and post on a particular newsgroup.

Using newsgroups varies depending on the way you are accessing the Internet. No matter whether you are using an on-line service, an Internet Service Provider, or just have access to a computer, the one piece of software you must have to use newgroups is a *newsreader.* A newsreader allows you to "subscribe" to and view newsgroups. Depending on the newsreader software, you will first have to "open" or "view" all the newsgroups before you can select the one or more you want to subscribe to. But be prepared — there are over 18,000 newsgroups to choose from! Once you have selected the newsgroup you want to subscribe to (don't worry subscribing is free and simply means selecting a newsgroup), you then need to retrieve the messages placed (or posted) on a particular newsgroup. Each of the commands to select, view, and retrieve new posts to a newsgroup is different in each newsreader, so you will need to become familiar with the particular newsreader you are using.

On-line service companies have the newsreader inherent in the software used to load their particular service. In this way, on-line services make it "easy" to find, read, and post to newgroups.

Using newsgroups is a bit more difficult if you use an Internet Service Provider and Web browser software. Although most of the newer browser software such as Netscape and Microsoft Explore contain newsreader software, your Internet Service Provider may only be subscribing to a particular number of newsgroups to save valuable space on their servers. For this reason, should you be unable to pull up a certain newsgroup, you may want to contact your Internet Service Provider and request that this newsgroup be added. Because newsgroups starting with "alt" (for alternative) tend to be topics which are sometimes controversial, your ISP might be holding it back on purpose. Again, try to contact your ISP to see if they will subscribe to the particular newsgroup you're requesting. The reason I mention this is that, sadly, many of the established infertility newsgroups begin with the "alt" prefix.

As a final note, if you just have access to a computer which does not have enough memory or disk space to load any of the fancy software to access the Internet, you can still load a plain newsreader application to access newsgroups. Check with your computer store for the best one for your existing system.

Some of the more popular newsgroups dealing with the whole realm of infertility include:

alt.infertility	discussion over whole range of infertility
alt.infertility.primary	support/discussion of individuals fighting primary infertility, and
misc.health.infertility	discussion on medical aspects of infertility

A complete listing of all the current newsgroups is in Appendix A.

BULLETIN BOARDS

Bulletin boards are basically the same as newsgroups, in the fact that they are a public place to post messages. However, they are much easier to use and do not require any additional software. Bulletin boards can be found on many Web sites and are also able on on-line service companies. On-line service companies might even refer to their bulletin boards as something different (such as America Online - which uses the term "message boards"). Nevertheless, they are another invaluable resource for information exchange.

As you read through and travel to some of the various Web sites listed in this book, you will notice many have their own bulletin boards covering all aspects of infertility and adoption. As an example, check out the many bulletin boards you can choose from at INCIID's site (www.inciid.org). In addition, instructions on how to find the specific infertility bulletin boards on America Online, are listed below:

America Online

➡ Click on Keyword

➡ Enter "pen" (without apostrophes)

➡ On the Personal Empowerment Network go down through the folders until you find: Reproduction & Infertility

➡ Double click on this — a menu of resources on infertility will come up. To view postings on infertility — click "Message Boards"

➡ Topic folders covering all aspects of infertility will pop up — to view any click on specific folder.

Other on-line service companies may also have similar boards dedicated to infertility or women's health issues, so you may want to investigate these if you are with another on-line service company.

CHAT ROOMS

I think the best aspect of chat rooms is this — they're fun! It's always fascinating to be able to type something on your terminal and automatically get a response from others. Many times you will find yourself in a chat room and someone will inevitably ask where everyone is from. It really gives you a sense of awe when you find out that some people in the chat are from Europe, Australia, or other parts of the globe and there they are — speaking with you live on-line!

There are many ways of chatting on-line with others on the topic of infertility. It is probably easiest, however, to use the ones available from the on-line service companies. An inherent part of any on-line service is their chat rooms. The respective topic bulletin boards often list where and when chats take place. For example, respective times for chats on infertility discussions will be mentioned in the folders on AOL's Personal Empowerment Network. When the specific time arrives all that's required is to go to the chat room. You automatically are able to join in the chat once you've entered the room.

If you are using a Internet Service Provider instead of an on-line service company, never fear — there are still ways for you to join in a live chat. As previously mentioned in Chapter 4, using the IRC - Internet Relay Chat is an option. You must have the software to be able to run this system, but accessing the software is free, and detailed instructions on how to do so are found on ONNA's Web site:

http://www.thought-crimes.com/onna

There are a couple other chat sites available on Web pages which I should mention. As of the time of this writing, neither is widely used but hopefully this will change as more people find out about them. The first is the Infertility Internet Chatsite:

http://www.uni.edu/~panak/iic.html

This site was created and is maintained by William Panak, PhD — an expert in infertility insurance coverage. Along with this chat site, an Adoption After Infertility chat site also exists and is linked from this page. Although it is hard to catch a large group of people in the chat site at one time an advantage that this site has over others is that it's self-archiving. What this means is that you can leave a question and check back within a day or two to see how people responded to your question.

Another previously mentioned Web site you can chat on is located at Fertile Thoughts:

http://www.bluestars.com/clinic/index.shtml

A couple of downsides of using chat rooms do exist, however. Since rooms sometimes do not carry a capacity limit, too many persons can cause the chats to become chaotic. (I've found this increasing true in the infertility chat rooms as people become more and more aware of this resource.) However, one way of getting around this is to move a particular conversation with a single individual into a private room — available on most public chat sites. The other side of this is that, on occasion, there will be so few people in the room that the momentum of the subject dies.

CHAPTER 6
MEDICAL INFO ON INFERTILITY

As you progress with your fertility treatments, you may want to find more information on the medications you are taking, or the latest advances in treating your diagnosis. The next two chapters will arm you with some excellent resources that are loaded with specific conditions and diagnoses.

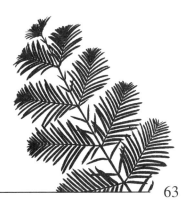

Atlanta Reproductive Health Centre

(http://www.ivf.com)

Atlanta Reproductive Health Centre WWW

Welcome to the Atlanta Reproductive Health Centre WWW homepage. You are one of 212106 visitors to this Webpage. It is my belief that properly informed, you can become an active participant in your healthcare and make better choices. My goal is to provide you with accurate information in areas of womens health including: infertility, IVF, endometriosis, contraception, sexually transmitted disease, menopause, stress management and PMS.

If you have installed RealAudio, you can listen to Dr. Perloe on Internet Radio.

ARHC Goes Shareware

The ARHC WWW has adopted the shareware concept. As this site has grown in popularity, it has become harder to respond to all questions. I spend a significant amount of time to review your background and your question and then attempt, respond appropriately. Please take a moment and consider what you have spent purchasing medical books and how much time, money and effort you might need to expend getting a simple question answered at your "offline" physician's office. By educating yourself and learning what questions to ask, you can enhance the value of your physician visit. Armed with the information contained in this WWW you can become a better healthcare consumer, achieve a more satisfactory result and save money. The Shareware means visit this site, take advantage of its many resources, if you find this site and the information you receive valuable, become an ARHC WWW Supporter by making a voluntary contribution.

As this WWW Homepage is a work in progress, your feedback is necessary to enable us to better meet your needs. Let us know if any of links from this page no longer work. And, if you have found this web site helpful, please tell your friends.

I mentioned previously that many infertility clinics have put themselves on the Web. Although many of these clinics do have some "shareable" information for most, their primary objective for having a presence on the Web is to recruit patients. However, it would be a crime not to spotlight the Atlanta Reproductive Health Centre in this book. The Web page was written and is maintained by Dr. Mark Perloe who truly understands the partnership that must be made between patient and doctor, particularly when it comes to infertility treatments. This Web page is a masterpiece and recieves awards on a regular basis. Not only is it informative, but Dr. Perloe has added the fun use of multimedia to make the learning experience more enjoyable.

Ever wonder why you sometimes you don't have a period? Or want to know exactly what endometriosis looks like? An invaluable freebie on this page is Miracle Babies — an entire on-line book written by Dr. Perloe and Linda Gail Christie. An excellent resource, Miracle Babies is a MUST READ for all persons in our shoes. Individual Chapters are listed on their own page and cover the entire gambit of diagnosis and treatment of infertility. This book answers questions that many of us have had for years and cannot find answers to anywhere else. The beautiful illustrations and pictures are an added bonus. Don't miss reading this in its entirety!

In addition to Miracle Babies, Dr. Perloe has loads of other specific information on his Web page. Stress, coping, PMS, pregnancy after infertility, reproductive surgery — you name it, it's probably somewhere on this page. You will find some of the latest-breaking information on the research side of infertility on this page, also. There is information on some of the latest male infertility treatment, on how extensive athleticism and eating disorders can impact your fertility, and on how previous diseases and cancer treatments can impair fertility. The amount of information available from this Web site cannot be adequately summarized in these couple pages. Therefore, I will mention that Dr. Perloe even included a "search" function to his site so that specifics can be identified. Say you want some information on fimbria deformities. After I entered the word "fimbria" in the search box I received five references on that particular topic alone!

One of the latest additions to this site is the ability to conference with Dr. Perloe about your particular situation *live!* Of course you will need some special teleconference capability with your computer, and you will also find that there is a fee attached to this service. Nevertheless, I'm sure many have found this service invaluable, especially after checking out and being impressed with his depth of knowledge through his Web site. I'm sure he has picked up a patient or two!

Serono

(http://www.serono-usa.com)

Anyone who has had the unfortunate chance of experiencing fertility drugs has certainly heard of Serono Laboratories. They are the makers of Fertinex™, Serophene™, and other well known fertility drugs. Specific information on their particular fertility drugs can be found on this site.

Serono Symposia USA, Inc.

(http://www.springer-ny.com/serosym/serono.htm)

Sponsored by Serono, Serono Symposia USA, Inc., is a nonprofit organization dedicated to the advancement of education in medicine. Frequently Serono Symposia offers grants to infertility support groups to aid in the increased knowledge of infertility causes and treatment of patients. The publications that Serono has to offer are geared toward medical professionals, as you will quickly see by the technicality and cost of the books. However, you may want to take advantage of some of them in your own research and, as previously mentioned, might be able to find them in a local medical library or by inquiring with your doctor who may lend them to you.

Mediconsult

(http://www.mediconsult.com)

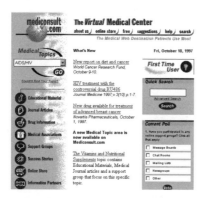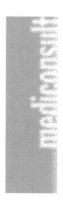

I literally fell upon this gem of a site while I was doing some research on pregnancy complications. Mediconsult is a Web service company which offers consultation on *all* types of medical conditions. Although not all of the company professionals are physicians, the information which the company uses to answer patients' questions comes from leading medical journals, medical conferences, pharmaceutical companies, and hospitals. On this main Web page you will notice dozens of medical conditions about which you can inquire. Of course, Infertility and Pregnancy Complications are two which you will want to peruse. Each topic leads to its own Web page where the following headings may be found:

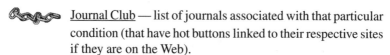 Journal Club — list of journals associated with that particular condition (that have hot buttons linked to their respective sites if they are on the Web).

Support Group — the main place you want to go to ask a question or find out answers to others questions.

Success Stories — what we all want to hear!

Educational Material — other magazines, support, etc.

Recommended Books

Drug Information — and it is searchable!

Mediconsult is probably the next best thing to asking a doctor directly. Credentials on the staff are listed on the home page and the service is free. Also keep in mind that the group pulls from a wide array of resources so that you have a *consensus* — not just one person's opinion regarding a condition or treatment.

American Society for Reproductive Medicine

(http://www.asrm.com)

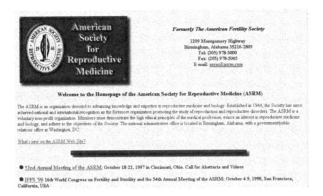

The American Society for Reproductive Medicine (ASRM) was founded in 1944 and is one of the oldest non-profit organizations in the field of reproduction. Its mission is to advance the knowledge and expertise of reproductive medicine. Only professionals in the field are allowed to be members of the ASRM, but the information that they hold, and much of what is on their Web page, is invaluable for all infertility patients. Some of the main features that you will want to check out include their Services Offered to Patients. Under this heading you will find:

 Frequently Asked Questions (about Infertility)

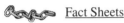 Fact Sheets

 Patient Information Series Booklets

ASRM's Fact Sheets (currently over a dozen available) cover a range of topics such as Counseling and Support: When and Where to Find It; Exercise, Weight, and Fertility; Intracytoplasmic Sperm Injection (ICSI); Multiple Gestation & Multifetal Pregnancy Reduction; Preimplantation Genetic Diagnosis; and Stress and Infertility — just to name a few. These are provided free of charge and are available on the Web site.

The Patient Information Series booklets are also invaluable resources but do cost $1.00 a piece (includes shipping.) Twice as many topics are covered, however, and in much more detail. Age & Infertility; Ectopic Pregnancy; Endometriosis; IVF & GIFT: A Guide to Assisted Reproductive Technologies; Miscarriage; and Uterine Fibroids are just several of the topics covered in the booklets.

The nice thing about both of these resources is that they are updated frequently.

ASRM is also the publisher of Fertility & Sterility — one of the foremost journals on reproduction. Although the subscription rate is most likely prohibitive for most of us (currently running $135/yr), the ASRM typically posts upcoming articles. This information is invaluable particularly if you have a nearby medical college. Most medical colleges allow public access to their libraries, where this journal (and many other related ones) are available. Take advantage of this opportunity if it exists for you!

Organon

(http://www.organon.nl)

Organon, another major pharaceutical company and makers of Humegon™ and Puregon™, also have a new presence on the Web. In addition to information about their products, Organon offers some useful Infertility facts.

Fertility Weekly

(http://www.homepage.holowww.com/1f.htm)

Fertility Weekly is a technical digest produced mainly for the medical field and contains some pretty specific articles on new tests and treatment on the fertility frontier. You can subscribe to this journal, but it is quite salty (currently $695/ yr.) However, it could be worth investigating merely for the technical information which it provides. On the home page you may find sample abstracts from some past editions of the digest. You may also order a Sample Request of the digest for free. Also check out a sample newsletter online located at:

http://www.newsfile.com/n_sample.htm

This page includes technical articles on topics such as sperm motility, lutenizing hormone, ectopic pregancy, and post-coital tests. If you are looking for some specific information on a condition or treatment you should give this site a visit.

Laparoscopy.com

(http://www.laparoscopy.com)

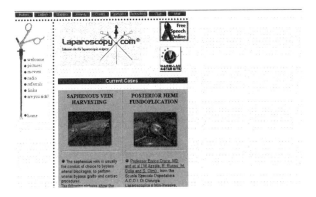

Laparoscopy has been used for a number of noninvasive surgeries — infertility diagnosis and treatment being just one of them. Dr. Alex Gandsas, a resident at North Oakland Medical Centers in Pontiac, Michigan has been fascinated himself with the endless possibilities in which Laparoscopy can be used, and decided to create this site in 1996 to share all which he has learned about the procedure.

Most of us who have been fighting infertility for some time have had (or are soon facing) a laparoscopy. As much as your doctor has told you about the procedure, you still might be a bit curious about it (especially if you are still facing this surgery). You can learn more about laparoscopy by taking advantage of this site. The site offers live conferences (via IRC chat) discussing laparoscopic surgery. Other information will be forthcoming such as a physician database for referrals. Live surgery demonstrations have already been performed and more are forecasted to take place in the future.

OBGYN.net

(http://www.obgyn.net)

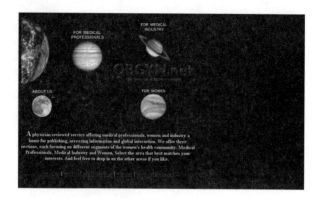

OBGYN.net is a wonderful international networking site constructed to be a forum for Ob/Gyn's and the women they serve. OBGYN.net allows practitioners and patients to meet and discuss women's health topics.

You may be able to learn some of the latest techniques and procedures in the Discussion bulletin boards under both the For Medical Professionals and For Women hyperlinks listed on their main home page. You can *subscribe* to the medical professional mail list, OB-GYN-L, but be advised you are only allowed to *post* to this group if you are a medical professional. (That's why they created the Women's Health section and discussion group, for patients to ask questions, and often doctors do reply to these postings.) Both lists are an excellent source for information and past discussion topics and can be searched by keyword, for example "infertility."

This site is so invaluable because of the availability to get information straight from the doctors themselves. Many of the doctors are involved on the board and some are even U.S. representatives — check out Our U.S. State Representatives under the About Us section on the home page.

The Journal of Obstetrics and Gynecology On-line

(http://www.ccspublishing.com/j_obg.htm)

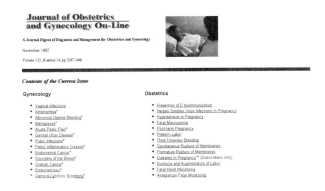

This journal, designed to encompass the whole realm of obstetrics and gynecology, contains topics of interest including <u>Amenorrhea</u>, <u>Endometriosis</u>, and <u>Infertility</u>. The only problem accessing parts of the journal is that they require you to download Acrobat Reader 3.0, which is available free to download from a link on this site. The program is fairly large (4 megabytes) and will take some time to download on-line (make sure to download the PDF version, since these files are PDF files.) However, once downloaded and installed, you may easily view the documents.

U of M Pathology Laboratory Handbook

(http://po.path.med.umich.edu/handbook/)

This is the University of Michigan Laboratory Handbook. At first glance, it may look a bit too technical but never fear! The best feature of this site is the *Find a Test in the Handbook* search tool. This is a wonderful resource for it shows not only a typical lab procedure for collection of the specimens, but also what the results should indicate. Want to know how long an estradiol sample should take, and what ranges they should fall within? Or how a beta hCG test is conducted? Or what progesterone levels should be in the first, second or third trimesters of pregnancy? You can find these values and more out simply by searching by using a keyword, such as hCG, estradiol, or progesterone. This resource is not just for fertility testing, so the whole gamut of medical tests can be found. And remember — this is one lab's interpretation — but it does fall in line with other information I have read elsewhere.

Chem-Tox: Researching Health Risks from Pesticides and Chemicals

(http://www.chem-tox.com)

Being a former environmental engineer myself, I feel I can say that much of the information regarding chemicals and their use has been over-emphasized by the media. I myself am very skeptical when I read any article that says we are being poisoned by the same chemicals which have improved our lifestyles significantly, and that the rise in infertility is primariliy being caused by overuse of chemicals. However, there still might be some truth to certain connections between use of certain chemicals and pesticides used *in the past* and their effects on one's fertility. For instance, the chemical Chlordane has been proven to cause serious health complications. You will find articles on this site linking pesticide and chemical use to various health concerns. A link to Infertility and Miscarriage Research Studies lists over 25 known facts about infertility and miscarriage and chemicals and cites their references. This site was created by a medical doctor, so much of the information and many of the references are legitimate. As always advised — use precaution in reviewing this information and try not to read too much into it.

The Merck Manual

(http://www.merck.com/!!rnvJG1RTtrnvJG1RTt/pubs/mmanual/)

The Merck Corporation is one of the world's largest pharmaceutical and health care companies. They have created a wonderful online resource in The Merck Manual. A comprehensive health guide, this manual is doubly impressive due to its easy-to-use searching feature. On the Manual's main page (listed above) you will find a search feature button where you can search and find very specific information on everything from "male infertility" to "PCO" to "ovarian failure."

Having problems with this challenging address? Then simply access the manual through their main Web page at www.merck.com.

National Institute of Child Health & Human Development

(http://web.fie.com/htdoc/fed/nih/nic/any/menu/any/nichd.htm)

The National Institute of Child Health & Human Development (NICHD) conducts and supports research on the reproductive and other processes that determine and maintain the health of children, adults, families and populations. Although this government organization has its own official Web page located at www.nih.gov/nichd, the address listed above is operated by FEDIX, a free online service which distributes information regarding federal grant money availability for participants in these studies. NICHD often grants money to couples who are willing to participate in new and innovative reproductive techniques. Some studies which NICHD has conducted in the past include research on preovarian failure, polycystic ovarian disease, and recurrent pregnancy loss.

Reuters Health Information Services

(http:// www.reutershealth.com)

Reuters Health Information Services is a wonderful research tool if you are looking for up-to-the-minute health news. Their site contains a powerful search tool which allows you to locate recent health related news articles on very specific subjects. After doing a recent search myself through this service I uncovered some real gems. Just as an exercise, try doing a simple search using the word "infertility." You'll be amazed at how many article summaries appear. However, in order to view these articles you must register with the service and obtain a user id and password.

healthfinder™

(http://www.healthfinder.gov)

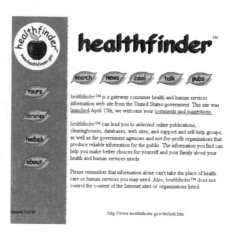

healthfinder™ (no, it is not capitalized) is a gateway consumer health and human services information Web site from the United States government. Some of the information available on this site is from governmental sources which have published their own studies. A three-way search function is available through this online service. The most valuable feature could be their alphabetical listing of health and human services topics. You will find many articles and other resources on infertility, pelvic inflammatory disease, and endometriosis, to name only a few findings under this search feature. When searching for "infertility" you will find a page on Infertility Services, a most helpful guide to understanding and comparing IVF clinic statistics.

CHAPTER 7

SPECIFIC DIAGNOSTIC WEB SITES

Once you've been diagnosed with a cause for your infertility, your natural reaction may be that you will want to learn as much as you can about that cause. I was surprised myself to find that such detailed information on specific diagnoses exists on the Web. Many of these Web pages were built by persons who have dealt with the diagnosis themselves and want to share information they have uncovered about their particular condition. Others are designed and operated by actual foundations or other nonprofit organizations.

MALE FACTOR

Being diagnosed with a severe male factor can be one of the biggest blows a couple experiences in life. For the man, it can completely annihilate his self-esteem. For the woman involved, hope can become a dim prospect. At this point in time, a couple which has been diagnosed with male factor usually has only two options — donor sperm or IVF with intracytoplasmic sperm injection (also known as ICSI). However, more is being learned each day as to the actual *causes* of male infertility which may provide future cures and options which are not currently available to a couple with this diagnosis. The first two sites listed below contain very specific information on male infertility and may aid you if you are dealing with this condition. Once again, we see where the Internet has become such a powerful tool in the fight against infertilty, as you will notice that both of the sites are international ones.

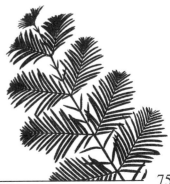

Spermatology

(http://numbat.murdoch.edu.au/spermatology/spermhp.html)

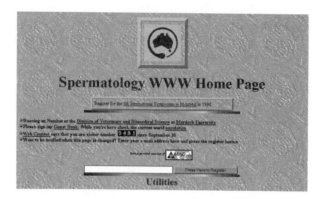

If you have been diagnosed with male factor infertility and feel hopeless, then make sure you don't miss this site! The site was developed by Dr. Jim Cummins who is an Associate Professor in Anatomy at Murdoch University in Australia.

The site contains some pretty heavy duty technical information so be fore-warned! However, there are several topics that you really should check out on this page. First off check out the Images of Sperm — neato! On this link you'll find loads of animal sperm images. This site also has one of the largest listings of Journals I've seen yet. As with all journals, they are expensive but wading through them might lead you to find a topic of interest. Under the Utilities and Monty Python link you'll find the Semen Analysis Handbook which was written as a lab manual but it is an excellent guide explaining how semen samples should be collected, handled, and analyzed. Another excellent resource is the Urology Database on Infertility, answering dozens of questions regarding male infertility. Also, the article Searching the Y chromosome for genes that cause infertility is particularly interesting. As should accompany all serious subjects, a bit of humor is provided under Every Sperm is Scared by Monty Python.

The Complete Urology, Andrology, & Male Infertility InfoBase

(http://platon.ee.duth.gr/~intermed/infobase/)

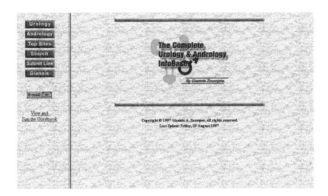

The Complete Urology & Andrology InfoBase is maintained by Giannis Zoumpos, MD, a research fellow at the Urologic Clinic of the Democritus University of Thrace, Greece. This international site provides some wonderful links to all sorts of Urology and Andrology resources. The difference between these two subsections of medicine is that *Urology* includes the study of the the urinary system in addition to the male reproductive system, whereas *Andrology* is a more specific study of only the male reproductive system. In either case, you will find Dedicated Sites, Associations, Journals, Personal Pages, Patient Oriented Pages, Support Groups, and Article links under both sources. A "don't miss" site if you are suffering from a male infertility diagnosis!

KLINEFELTERS SYNDROME

A serious form of male infertility can be caused by Klinefelters Syndrome. This condition is cause by a variation in the sex chromosomes in men. Men are made up of a X and a Y chromosome. With this condition, however, one or more X chromosomes combine at conception to cause varying degrees of complications to the male offspring. Males with Klinefelters Syndrome often are infertile, have learning disabilities, have enlarged breasts and/or are of small or incomplete masculine build. Once again, the symptoms vary but many men respond well to testosterone therapy, due to the fact that this is primarily a hormonal disease.

Klinefelters Syndrome

(http://www.genetic.org/ks/)

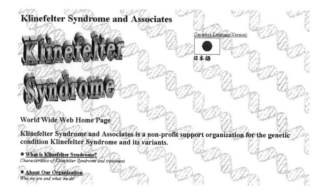

Klinefelters Syndrome is a nonprofit organization started in 1989 by Melissa Aylstock who, as a mother, started the organization to raise awareness about this condition. The organization helps promote research for Klinefelters Syndrome and publishes a newsletter three times a year to its members. You may view Past Newsletters on their home page. This well laid out Web page also includes information on What is Klinefelters Syndrome as well as Klinefelters Research Projects and Interesting Press Releases.

DES

If you've been diagnosed with a T-shaped uterus or have a "hooded" cervix then you probably know that such structural changes are usually the result of exposure to DES. DES (diethylstilbestrol) was a common drug given to pregnant women between 1938-1971 to prevent miscarriages. However, this well intentioned drug caused some serious health problems for the offspring of pregnant women who took it. It has been know to cause a rare cancer of the vagina or cervix in female offspring of women who were prescribed DES. All offspring (men as well as women) also often suffer from reproductive problems as well.

There are several Web sites which offer support and information for those suffering with DES exposure.

DES Action USA

(http://www.desaction.org)

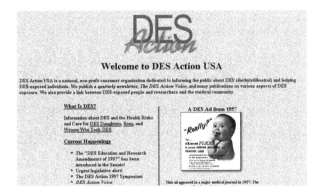

DES Action was founded in 1977. Services offered by DES Action include a quarterly newsletter, low cost publications, physician and attorney referral lists, advocacy, and a member hotline. See their Web page on ways of finding out if you could have been exposed to DES. Also check out their Frequently Asked Questions about DES.

DES Daughters

(http://www.surrogacy.com/online_support/des/)

This Web site was created by TASC (see Chapter 8) and basically serves as a quick access route to TASC's own mailing list for women suffering from DES. The mailing list is highly confidential and requires a password to enter the group. TASC has also established a Chat room specifically for DES Daughters where physicians, attorneys and psychologists are often guest speakers.

Professor Sally's DES Page

(http://www.geocities.com/HotSprings/2510/)

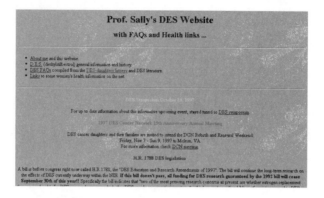

Professor Sally Glover is not a medical doctor but does have her doctorate in Mathematics. Her expertise, however, has also expanded to DES — having been personally affected by the drug. She has put together her own Web page which contains a collection of information that she has acquired from newsgroups and the DES-daughter's mailing list, which she co-moderates. Make sure you check out her general information on <u>DES,</u> as well as <u>DES FAQs.</u>

ENDOMETRIOSIS

If you are one of the many women suffering from endometriosis then you know how frustrating (and often painful) the disease is. Although endometriosis is the number one cause of infertility in women, no known cause or cure has yet been found. There is an national Endometriosis Association but, as of this writing, they do not currently have a Web Page. However, be sure not to miss the subpage of the Atlanta Reproductive Health Centre (see Chapter 6) on Overcoming Endometriosis. You can find this page directly at:

http://www.ivf.com/endohtml.html

The following Web sites also hold loads of information which might help with your studying.

Endometriosis Resources

(http://www.geocities.com/Hotsprings/1712/endo.htm)

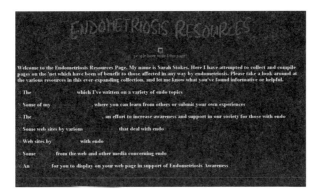

This Web site was created and maintained by a young woman named Sarah Stokes, who was only 11 when she began having symptoms of her endometriosis. Her story illustrates how this illness can affect a women of any childbearing age. This is one of the most comprehensive endometriosis Web pages I have found on the subject. In addition to the endometriosis Web pages discussed in this section, other links on this site include:

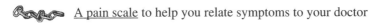 A pain scale to help you relate symptoms to your doctor

A page about Pain Management (self-authored)

Some General Information about Endometriosis (by the Mental Health Net)

Some information about the Treatment of Endometriosis

A Quick guide to joining the WINSENDO mailing list

Other personal endometriosis web pages

Endometriosis by Ari Babaknia, MD

(http://www.bioscience.org/books/endomet/babaknia.htm)

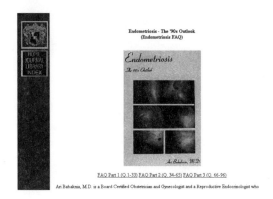

Available through Frontiers in Bioscience (an on-line nonprofit journal of broad biomedical topics, human reproduction being just one) this book on endometriosis is unique in that it is put together in a question and answer format. Close to 100 questions regarding endometriosis are answered in depth by its author, Ari Babaknia, MD. Be sure to also check out Frontiers in Bioscience's home page at:

www.bioscience.org

for other fertility-related journal articles.

TV Documentary in Production on Endometriosis

(http://www.endometriosis.org)

This is a unique Web page for it is being used to gather information (and funding) for its production of *Waiting for a Cure* — an hour long TV documentary on endometriosis. The film is being produced by the University of Texas Science Center at San Antonio which is a non-profit group dedicated to the advancement of medical research and education. This page lays out some of the information they have already collected for their documentary and includes:

- What is it?
- What does it look like?
- Theoretical causes
- Symptoms
- Myths about endometriosis
- Treatment Options
- Interview with Women with Endometriosis and Medical Experts

POLYCYSTIC OVARIAN SYNDROME (PCOS)

Also known as Hyperandrogenic Anovulation or Stein-Leventhal Syndrome, PCO is a disease which causes the ovaries to become covered with cysts due to an imbalance of hormones. Normally PCO manifests itself with symptoms including excessive weight gain, facial hair, acne, and greasy skin. Because of the hormonal imbalance, PCO also manifests itself by scant or absent periods and the inability to conceive.

PCO sufferers finally have a formal association — being formed through PCO Support — so be sure to check it out. If you are suffering from PCO, the following Web site may also be of value to you:

http://www.best.com/~mclark/pco

This is a collection of archived letters from the PCO mailing list. You may at least be able to find an e-mail buddy by wading through all the messages.

PCO Support —
Polycystic Ovarian Syndrome Association

(http://www.pcosupport.org)

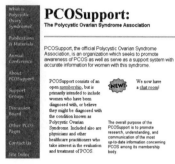

Recently founded, PCOSupport strives to be your sole source for PCO information and support. Membership in the association is $30 and chapters are currently forming throughout the United States. Selected Medical Journal Articles, Symptoms & Associated Health Risks and Treatments & Medications are some of the resources available under their What is Polycystic Ovary Syndrome? link.

In addition to the large amount of information they provide, many support options exist on their site. You can choose participation in their Chat Room, links to other Support Groups, or posting to others via their Discussion Board. Links to Other PCOS Pages abound on the site, as well.

TURNER'S SYNDROME

Turner's syndrome is basically the female counterpart to Klinefelter's syndrome. Like KS, Turner's syndrome is a chromosomal condition. However, Turner's syndrome appears in females and is caused by the complete or partial lack of one of the X chromosomes which makes up a woman. This lack of an X chromosome manifests itself in the female by causing infertility and short stature. In addition, other health conditions could result such as heart, kidney, or thyroid problems.

The Turner's Syndrome Society of the United States

(http://www.turner-syndrome-us.org)

Founded in 1987, the Turner's Syndrome Society now contains over 36 chapters nationwide. Like the Klinefelter organization, the Turner's Syndrome Society publishes a quarterly newsletter to its members. Selections from it can be found on their main Web page. There you will also find good links to Frequently Asked Questions about Turner's Syndrome and Publications Available from the Society. If you are affected by this condition, there also is a place for you to post for an online penpal under the Cyber Chapter of TSS to share information. A Chat Room is also available for ongoing conversation and scheduled forums on the subject.

LUPRON

Lupron has been used in the medical field for many years for many conditions. In infertility, it is often used prior to an IVF cycle to suppress a woman's hormones so that when the fertility drugs are given her system will respond better. It has also been used in some cases to reduce the effects of endometriosis. However, Lupron, like many other drugs, carries some possible side effects with it. Although most women have not experienced these effects, some women have, and here is a resource where you can read about some of these possible side effects. Remember, after all, that even some well-intentioned drugs of the past have often been found to have extreme side effects — look at DES, for example. I debated whether to put this site in this book, but thought it may be of value to some. Please approach it with caution and always ask your doctor to cross-reference what you read. Remember, however, that ultimately it is your body!

The National Lupron Victims Network

(http://www.voicenet.com/~nlvn/)

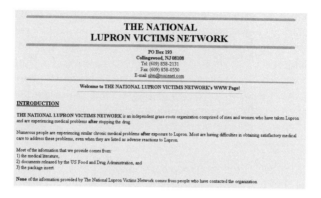

Founded in 1994 by Dr. Linda Abend, the National Lupron Victims Network is a grassroots organization of men and women who have used Lupron in the past, some of which are now experiencing medical side effects from the drug. Apparently the information laid out in the site is cited from medical literature and FDA documents. Some of the many reports listed on their site include:

- Lupron: Adverse Reactions (Men, Women, & Children)

- Lupron: Never Approved for Infertility Treatment

- Lupron: Endometriosis

- Lupron: Autoimmune Disorders and an Effect on the Immune System

- Lupron: Does Lupron Put You Into Menopause ?

and many, many, more.

CHAPTER 8
ALTERNATIVE METHODS

Although it is highly debated, some alternative methods claim to have succeeded in helping some women become pregnant and carry their babies to term. Western science often tends to discount these alternatives, and most of the time they should be skeptical in doing so. After all, infertility is often caused by structural deformations, which only science and a trained reproductive surgeon may be able to fix. However, especially when you are dealing with hormonal problems or unknown factors, the use of herbs or other homeopathic therapies may contribute to successful results.

You may or may not want to try to use any of these natural methods. What may work for another person may have no effect at all on you. However, most of these methods are harmless, and they may at least relax you and give you some extra peace in your life (especially from the hectic tests and treatments). But once again, I urge you to be a wise consumer of the information you find on these Web sites. Remember that there is no magical formula to cure infertility — no matter who hypes it. And, as always, you should consult with your fertility specialist as to the risks involved in using any of these methods.

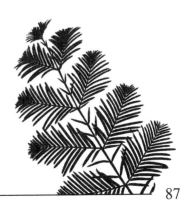

Acupuncture.com

(http://www.acupuncture.com)

For thousands of years, acupuncture has been one of the common practices of Chinese medicine. It involves insertion of very thin needles into parts of the body which are then supposed to release an energy known as Qi (pronounced chee). Although Acupuncture is this site's name, this Web page presents a good overview of Traditional Chinese Medicine (TCM) in general. Under the Acupuncture link you will find a link to its use in Infertility. In addition to how acupuncture works, you will find an in-depth look at Chinese herbs by linking to the Herbology page. Under this link you will find an article on Male Infertility and a Discussion of Spermophlebectasia. Back on the home page, if you are interested in pursuing use of these methods, you may find a therapist in your area in the Practioner List. Still skeptical? Then make sure to read some of the Treatment Testemonials.

American Alliance of Aromatherapy

(http://www.healthy.net/pan/pa/Aromatherapy/aaat/)

The technique of aromatherapy uses highly concentrated extracts of flowers and plants, known as essential oils, as a means to heal. The use of these oils may be administered by diffusers, baths, or in some case, direct application. The American Alliance of Aromatherapy is a nonprofit organization whose mission is to promote the use of aromatherapy as alternative treatment. On this site you will find information About the American Alliance of Aromatherapy. Although this organization seems to be in its infancy, you can find out more about aromatherapy in general by subscribing to The International Journal of Aromatherpy found on their site.

American Yoga Association

(http://members.aol.com/amyogaassn/)

Yoga combines stretching, breathing, meditation, and often chanting in its attempt to bring relaxation and healing to the person who is performing it. Like many of these natural methods, there are numerous sites on the Internet to get information on yoga. A quick search will unveil tons of resources on this subject alone. However, by visiting this one site you will be able to find out What is Yoga, The Techniques of Yoga, and the Yoga Philosophy.

Home of Reflexology

(http://www.reflexology.org)

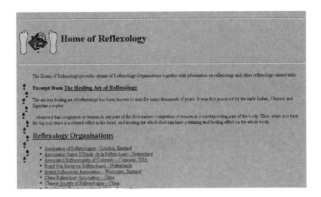

My philosophy on reflexology is this — if it involves a foot message and will relax me — I'm all for it! Even if it proves not to cure my infertility, it's a definite stress reducer. It's sometimes difficult to locate books written on reflexology so these next couple of sites may be able to add to your knowledge of it. On this page you will find numerous hyperlinks to other organizations and associations throughout the world under the Reflexology Organisations heading. As you might be able to tell once viewing this site, it is an international one. The Healing Art of Reflexology details what reflexology is and how it works. For more information on reflexology, check out the Reflexology Related Links.

YogaClass.com

(http://www.yogaclass.com)

If your interested in yoga after visiting the American Yoga Association, why not try out a bit by visiting YogaClass.com? This is an online self-instructional interactive site where you are given step-by-step instructions on how to do yoga. By visiting YogaCentral you may learn the various yoga techniques including a workout, breathing, relaxation and chanting. Under the YogaClass Links you will find articles such as Is Yoga unChristian? and Yoga for HIV Management.

Reflexology Research

(http://www.reflexology-research.com)

Where and how did the practice of Reflexology get started? The heading Definition and Brief History of Reflexology will answer that question. Technical aspects of reflexology are discussed on the home page. If you are still cynical, then browse the link to a Review-Analysis of the Effectiveness of Foot Reflexology Applied to 8,096 Clinical cases. And, if you want to find out how reflexology can help infertility, look under the A-Z Research list.

Reflexology Research even publishes a journal Reflexions to which you can subscribe on this page. If you still desire to find out more information on this topic, here is one of the few places where you can purchase one of their Reflexology Books in Print.

Moonrise Herbs

(http://www.moonrise.botanical.com/index2.html)

Moonrise Herbs also is a company and, much like Herbal Resources, it's listed here due to some of the good information and products it offers on its page. For more information on herbs, there is a link to Botanical.com. On the Botanical.com page you will find information on herbs under the Modern Herbal hyperlink. Over 800 herbs are listed in this directory.

Back on the Moonrise Herb page you will find another link to Intimacy & Conception. This is one of my personal favorites, for it offers some products to help keep the spark alive between the two of you while you try to conceive that baby. In addition to some conception teas you will find sensual bath oils, soaps, and massage oils. Many books can be also purchased on how to administer massages and keep that romantic flame burning brightly. You may also order Herbs and essential oils used in Aromatherapy from this company.

Homeopathy Home Page

(http://www.dungeon.com/~cam/)

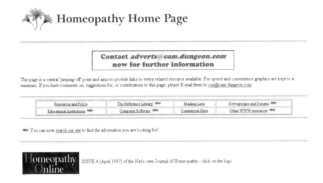

Homeopathy began in the 19th century and has had a resurgence in the last 15 years as an alternative medicine practice. Homeopathy uses small single doses of a medicine which has been shown to cause the same symptoms as the person is experiencing with their illness.

This Web page was created in the United Kingdom by Bernie Simon who has successfully used homeopathy to cure the aches and pains encountered due to his involvement in the martial arts. This site is really just a well laid out set of hyperlinks to resources dealing with homeopathy. You can access the online journal Homeopathy Online as well as subscribe to the Homeopathy Mailing List and Holistic Discussion Group easily from his home page. In addition, you can find links to the National Center for Homeopathy and the American Association of Naturopathic Physicians under the U.S.A. Addresses link. Both services will help you locate practicing physicians in your area.

Holistic Healing Web Page

(http://www.holisticmed.com)

Although not very fancy, the Holistic Healing Web page is another great hyperlink page. Many resources to holistic medicine can be found on this page including a huge listing of alternative newsgroups and mailing lists. Megalinks on how to Find a Holistic Practitioner can also be found on the main Web page. Many other links to Acupuncture, Aromatherapy, Chiropractic, Herbalism, Homeopathy, Naturopathic Medicine, Oriental Medicine, and Yoga can be found though this site.

Herbal Resources Inc.

(http://www.herbsinfo.com)

Herbal Resources Inc.'s site contains some interesting information under its Clinical Research Bulletins hyperlink. Here you may find loads of information on exactly how specific herbs aid in helping relieve PMS and curing luteal phase defects. This extensive article also offers some suggestions on how to relieve PMS though use of vitamins and lifestyle changes. On the Home page, you will also be able to learn A Short History of Herbs as well as How to Prepare and Use Herbs. And, of course, you may order Herbs through this company.

Algy's Herb page - Apothecary

(http://www.algy.com/herb/medcat.html)

Algy's Herb page is an extremely comprehensive herb resource. Although containing many links to other sites, you will want to make a stop at this site if you are interested in possible herbal remedies for your infertility, since the designer of this site has neatly organized these links into appropriate subject catagories. There is "must read" information under the *Caution* section of herbal uses. Some all-around information on herbs can be found under the *Basics* subheading. Finally, you can learn some ways of preparing herbs under the *Preparation* section.

Herbal Materia Medica

(http://www.healthy.net/clinic/therapy/herbal/herbic/herbs/)

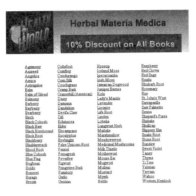

If you're looking for an excellent herbal resource, then you must check out Herbal Materia Medica. One of the many resources offered by Health World Online, this particular site contains a comprehensive herbal directory, including illustrations and extensive information on over 150 different herbs. Here you will find reviews on some of the herbs claimed to increase fertility such as Chaste Berry, False Unicorn Root, Raspberry, and Wild Yam.

As previously mentioned, this resource is part of a larger site — Health World Online (http://www.healthy.net), which you will also want to investigate in it's entirety. Founded by partners, President Dave Robertson and Vice President Jim Strohecker, Health World's mission is to provide what they have dubbed Self-Managed Care™ — a forum which allows people to manage their own health. And as you will see, you can find a tremendous amount of information on all forms of natural healing methods on this vast site. Make sure not to miss the many Infertility related articles under their Diseases & Conditions link. Additional natural methods may be found under their Alternative Therapies listing, as well.

Mother Nature's General Store

(http://www.mothernature.com)

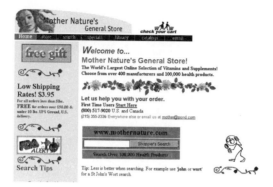

One last company I must mention is Mother Nature's General Store. By clicking on the link to the actual store itself, you will find yet another extensive listing of information on <u>Herbs,</u> in addition to some other resources such as <u>Massage Oils, Aromatherapy,</u> <u>Herbal Teas</u>, and <u>Vitamin & Supplements</u>. And be sure not to miss the resource for <u>Better Sex Through Vitamins and Natural Foods</u>. Under this hyperlink, you will find information on vitamins, herbs, and foods which have been known to help improve the libido and reproductive system. You may find resources to purchasing each product under its appropriate link.

Fertile Ground Network

(http://www.tiac.net/users/fertile)

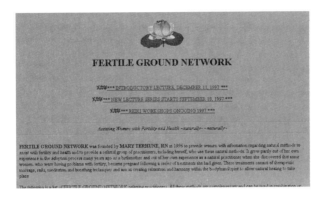

OK, folks, this is the last site I'll feature in this chapter, and it's about as "new age" as you can get. The Fertile Ground Network was founded in 1996 by Mary Terhune, RN. She is a Reiki Master, Certified Muscular Therapist and Meditation Teacher. Through the use of these techniques, she believes a woman increases her chances at conceiving.

There are five other instructors which are a part of the Fertile Ground Network. Joan Ruggier also offers Reiki Workshops. (Reiki apparently is a non-invasive hands-on healing technique which uses the energy in your body to reduce stress.) Patricia Racholwski operates her business Full Cycle which teaches women how to use herbs to help regulate a woman's reproductive cycle. Mary Finnegan owns the Fertility Awareness Services which teaches the natural methods of birth control and increasing your chances of conception through the knowledge of your own body's fertility signs.

Perhaps the two most unusual conception methods are taught by Janice Cummings and Cheryl Procaccini. Cheryl Procaccini uses Medicine Song which is a sound therapy used to release energy from your body to treat and heal imbalances in it. Janice Cummings operates the Cosmic Order Studio and practices cosmobiology which is the study of the effect of the planets on the biological systems of Earth.

CHAPTER 9
GRIEF / ADDITIONAL LOSS SUPPORT SITES

Having been dealt this painful infertility card in life, those of us suffering from it can attest that we eventually realize that life is not fair. Unfortunately for some, life can get even crueler at times. Not only are some people faced with infertility, but after finally "conquering" it with a pregnancy, some people sometimes experience additional losses through miscarriage, stillbirth, selective reduction, or pregnancy termination due to ectopic pregnancies or fetal deformities. The following Web sites deal with these difficult, trying, and heartbreaking times. They were written by people who have experienced multiple losses and may become one of your greatest support mechanisms if you have also experience such losses. As far away as it may seem, hope and living can return with time. Maybe a visit to these sites will aid with your grief.

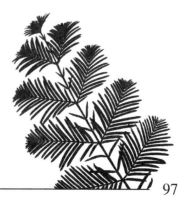

Miscarriage by Dawn Banks George

(http://www.hcc.cc.fl.us/services/staff/dawn/miscarry.htm)

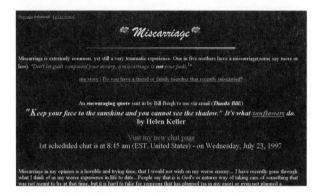

Persons suffering from miscarriages often suffer alone. This usually happens because society normally does not recognize the pregnancy for what it was — a human life which has been lost. Even pro-choice believers can certainly understand that at least a loss exists. And this loss is often further not recognized by relatives and friends because there is no formal closure to the ordeal. When a person dies, a ceremony (the funeral) helps us to move forward in the grieving process. But when a miscarriage happens, often there is not the opportunity for a funeral or to say good-bye.

Having suffered from a miscarriage herself, Dawn Banks George designed her page to help others with pregnancy loss and to show them that they were not alone. Once again, it is a wonderful example of how one person can make something good happen out of a terrible experience. While listening to inspiring music on her page you can visit her <u>Chat room</u> for miscarriage support or link one of the many sites she has collected on miscarriage information. These include everything from general <u>Questions and Answers about Miscarriage</u> to many other technical articles discussing miscarriage from reliable sources such as clinic pages and doctors. Help others understand your situation by giving them the link to <u>Do you have a friend or family member that recently miscarried?</u> And be sure to take advantage of her <u>Happy Thoughts and Favorite Things</u> link.

Toni's Angel Pages in Support of Pregnancy

(http://www.geocities.com/Heartland/8242/)

Toni's Angel Pages is dedicated to the whole realm of pregnancy and the potential losses which often exist with it. As well as many links she has collected on Pregnancy and Pregnancy Loss, there are also links to Infertility and Health. Be sure not to miss her Stories from the Heart, where others have posted their stories of loss; you can do so as well if you so wish. (Note: In the process of editing this book, the author of this Web site mysteriously vanished and a police investigation was underway as to her disappearance. Information on this tragic event is posted on this page.)

The Miscarriage Page

(http://teramonger.com/dwan/html/Miscpage.htm)

This is also an incredibly informative Web site which may help you in your grief. It offers not only support but information which may help you in the future to prevent further losses. Dwan Tape, the creator of the site, has collected information specifically on miscarriage from many of the resources I have already covered in this book. However, she has put them together as easily accessible links on this well-organized Web site. Some of her links include Books and Other Resources, General Information/Articles, How to Help (a guide for family/friends to help the person who has gone through a miscarriage), Possible Reasons or Causes, and Prevention Possibilities.

Christian Pregnancy Loss Support

(http://www.geocities.com/Wellesley/2458/)

For those of you who are looking for Christian pregnancy loss support pages here is another resource in addition to Hannah's Prayer, reviewed in Chapter 4. Christian Pregnancy Loss Support began as a mailing list and grew to have its own Web site. On the site you will find out how to join the mailing list under Subscription Information. There are also a growing number of Inspirational Poems and members' stories listed on this site. And, since it is a Christian site, a Prayer Request and Comment link is provided for your use.

A Heartbreaking Choice

(http://www.erichad.com/ahc/)

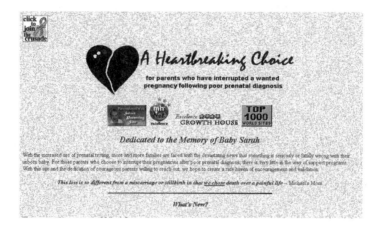

So you finally got pregnant and you anxiously go in to your doctor for a regular checkup. After some prenatal testing, he/she informs you that there is something seriously or fatally wrong with your child. What do you do? For some parents a choice is made to terminate the pregnancy, believing that death is better than a painful life for the child. In some cases, death for the child is imminent. In any case, this site is appropriately named. On-line chats and a mailing list for parents in this situation are available through this Web site. A visit to A Heartbreaking Choice may aid you with your decision if you are in this terrifying position.

SANDS

(http://www.vicnet.net.au/~sands/sands.htm)

Originating in Victoria, Australia, this site attests to the invaluable nature of the Internet. Stillbirth and Neonatal Death Support (SANDS) is a support group for parents who have experienced these losses (including miscarriage.) It contains some of the most helpful information on loss and grieving. The Dedication Wall is particularly endearing. Parents who have lost children may post their own dedication to their child on this page. Other helpful coping mechanisms are also provided, including suggestions on how to grieve for your baby, and moving through your grief and on with life. Audio Files & Multimedia on coping strategies and grieving also may also be useful to you. Many other good links exist to other grief, bereavement and medical resource sites.

Hygeia™

(An Online Journal for Pregnancy and Neonatal Loss)

(http://www.hygeia.org)

Just as despair can come to one only from other human beings,
Hope, too, can come to one only from other human beings.
Elie Wiesel

Continue

If you are grieving, you *must* visit this site. Created and maintained by Michael R. Berman, MD, Hygeia™ is an excellent on-line support mechanism for those who are suffering from pregnancy or neonatal loss. On the <u>Index</u> page you will find aspects of loss discussed from different perspectives in <u>The Journal</u> link. Each journal topic is beautifully forwarded by a poem expressing that aspect of loss. In addition to these poems, others may be found on the Index in <u>The Poems</u> section. These poems are composed by Dr. Berman, himself, who wrote them for his patients who had miscarried. Sharing of visitors' loss experiences may be found in <u>Visitors' Stories.</u> You may also join in the discussion with others on the site when you <u>Register as a User</u>. Reading through much of the stories and emotions on this site is heart-wrenching, but I'm sure it will be sincerely comforting to those who also have experienced the same types of losses.

Abiding Hearts

(http://www.asfhelp.com/AHTOC.HTM)

Abiding Hearts is a nonprofit organization dedicated to aiding those who wish to continue their pregnancies even though a pre-natal test has revealed fatal or non-fatal birth defects of the baby. Although very simple, the site offers valuable support through lists of <u>Suggested Reading</u>, <u>Music to Listen to</u>, and the <u>Parent's Bill of Rights</u>. There also is a <u>Sample Delivery Wish List</u> for the parents who have decided to go to term, as well as ways friends and family can help the couple cope with their tough decision through the long months ahead.

GriefNet

(http://rivendell.org)

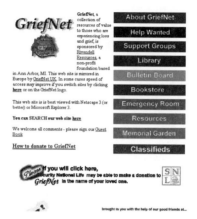

Founded by Cendra Lynn, a psychologist in Ann Arbor, Michigan, GriefNet has become an on-line international safety net for those mourning all types of losses. Developed in 1994, GriefNet is an electronic extension of Rivendell Resources — a non-profit grief resources organization providing workshops and counselling — which Cendra incorporated in 1992. Run by a volunteer staff of over sixty people around the world, GriefNet is funded by donations, Classified Advertising, its Bookstore, and underwriting.

GriefNet's Support Groups are run through an email system which you may easily join, and are specific and wide ranging. Not only will you find a support group for neonatal loss, but for sibling, parent, and even pet losses. (I lost my dog in the midst of our infertility struggle and I thought I was going to die myself. At the time I was sure it was a sign from God that I wasn't even fit to take care of a dog, little alone be a mother! Strange things your mind can make you think when in the mist of grief.) Some of the information in their Library consists of Articles and Manuscripts, Books, Poetry, and Thoughts and Ideas, and an Annotated Bibliograpy in the making. And the Memorial Garden is a lovely place to make a special dedication to the one you miss and love so much.

CHAPTER 10
Finding Resolution

As I have learned over my many years of battling infertility, success in overcoming infertility can come in many forms. For those just starting on their journey, some of the options laid out in this chapter may seem unimaginable now. However, as many of us who have come through this process can attest, peace of mind and heart may eventually be found through embracing one or more of these options. Additional support, both emotional and informational, is a necessity if you are considering any of them.

SURROGACY

Surrogacy comes in many forms. Classically, surrogacy has been perceived as a third party carrying the embryo of an infertile couple. However, the definition also includes sperm donation and egg donation. Moving forward toward this option brings along its own challenges — including additional legal and financial aspects, just to name a couple. The Internet provides several excellent resources to help you investigate surrogacy, make an informed decision, and possibly even find a surrogate.

If you happen to live in the United Kingdom — make sure you check out Childless Overcome Through Surrogacy (COTS) located at:

www.netlink.co.uk/users/cots

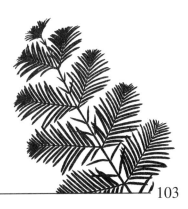

The American Surrogacy Center, Inc. (TASC)

(http://www.surrogacy.com)

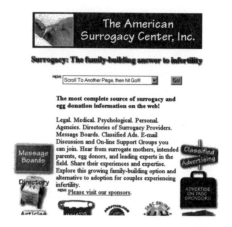

The American Surrogacy Center (TASC) was founded by Joan Barnes who herself has had two children successfully through surrogacy. TASC is one of the best resources for original information regarding surrogacy. By clicking on message boards, TASC lays out over a dozen topics in a unique interactive question and answer format. You can post a question, and either a professional or other person who has had experience with the topic will reply. Some of these include:

- Is the Doctor In? — Medical Q & A

- Is the Lawyer In? — Legal Q & A

- Is the Agency In? — Agencies and people who have used them

- Financial Discussion — Q & A on all costs involved

- Insurance Questions & Dilemmas — How Surrogacy further complicates this matter

- Gestational Surrogacy, Egg Donation, Traditional-AI Surrogacy — Q & A with others who have undergone these treatments

If you are trying to locate a doctor, lawyer, or agency in your state to help with surrogacy, click on the Directory. Support Groups and Related Links are also listed under the Directory, so make sure you don't miss some of these valuable

Internet links. Click on Articles for additional information on the medical, legal, and agency aspects. Personal Stories, also found in the Article section, give accounts of success through surrogacy.

TASC also offers on-line seminars and an on-line newsletter which is filled with tons of information. The Surrogacy Store® is filled with additional books, videos, and inspirational gifts which may be purchased.

Most of all, if you believe surrogacy is for you and want to start searching for a potential surrogate, that, too, is offered on this site. Under the Classified Advertising, you may be able to identify an egg or sperm donor, or a third-party surrogate.

Organization of Parents through Surrogacy (OPTS)

(http://www.opts.com)

The Organization of Parents Through Surrogacy

Information -- Education -- Networking

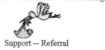

Support -- Referral

     The Organization of Parents through Surrogacy (OPTS) is an independent, non-commercial, informational, and advocacy organization for families built through surrogate parenting. The group has an active phone and on-line member network and has an annual newsletter. It also has regional meetings for members. Legal, medical, psychological, and agency/clinic resources are included with membership, as well as legislative updates. Their Web site presence continues to grow. You can join this organization on-line and receive these invaluable resources offered through membership.

Surrogate Mothers Online

(http://www.geocities.com/Wellesley/2025)

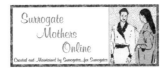

Welcome to the Surrogate Mothers Online home page! Our purpose is to provide information, support, and friendship to surrogate mothers and potential surrogate mothers. Parents and prospective parents via surrogacy are, of course, welcome to visit and participate as well!

We invite you to browse through the information we have compiled. We hope it will be a helpful resource to you! If you are interested, you might also like to read or post to our surrogacy message board or our classified section. Please keep in mind that we are still under construction and pardon our dust for the moment. There will be lots of new material coming soon so we hope you will keep checking back!!!

GREAT NEWS!!! We are pleased to announce that the classified section, message board and guestbook are all working once again. We have moved them to a new server in hopes that it will be more reliable than the last one.

Unfortunately, the most recently posted messages and ads, placed during the last few days on the old server, have been lost. If you posted a message recently and you cannot find it, please accept our sincerest apology and feel free to repost, any time. :o)

Articles

We are currently in the process of collecting articles about a wide range of surrogacy topics, including how to decide if surrogacy is

Surrogate Mothers Online came online in 1997 and offers more information on surrogacy. On this site, you will find a large array of surrogacy articles. A bulletin board is also available, where you may correspond with others about surrogacy experiences. And don't miss the FREE Virtual Classifieds for Surrogacy, Egg/Sperm Donation and Adoption. These classified contains a wide range of services pertaining to potential surrogates, donors, adoptive parents, and birth parents. Since the site has just recently come online, I'd expect more expansion of this Web page in the future.

Surrogate Mothers, Inc.

(http://www.surrogatemothers.com)

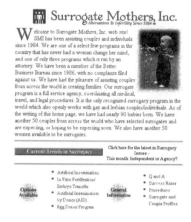

Surrogate Mothers, Inc. is actually an agency but is listed here because it contains some valuable information most other on-line surrogacy agencies do not provide. General Information lays out some frequently asked questions. Approximate Expenses and Legal Issues are "don't miss" links to visit if you are pursuing this option.

ADOPTION

Fortunately there are so many resources on the Internet for adoption that I could probably write a book on it alone. However, I have just listed some of my top picks in this section. If you are considering adoption (or in the process of adopting), then you will soon find out (or already know) what a rollercoaster itself it can be. As with infertility, adoption opens up a whole other can of considerations. Should we go through an agency? Should we independently adopt? What about international adoption? Could we adopt a special needs child?

My husband and I have explored every one of these options — and each has its own advantages and disadvantages. As with going through infertility treatment, you must be informed about adoption to be able to make the best decision for yourself and the child. After you investigate these sites, you may also want to do an additional search on adoption to find more information. Many adoption agencies are now on-line. Unlike the list of infertility clinics located in Appendix B, I will let you do the searching for most of these. However, I have included a few in this section to give you a flavor of the services they offer.

Adoption.com

(http://www.adoption.com)

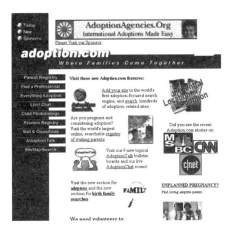

Gee, that one is sort of easy to remember! And if you are going through or considering adoption, it's good that it is — for you will definitely not want to miss this site. This site was created by Nathan Gwilliam, the President and CEO of Adoption.com. After spending some time in Brazil a few years ago, he realized that there was still a need for good international adoption agencies and of general adoption information. When the Internet became such a hit, he quickly recognized it as an excellent resource for his agency to bring families together.

This site offers many invaluable opportunities and resources Birthmothers and agencies may identify potential parents through Adoptive Parents Registry, on which couples seeking to adopt may purchase a listing to advertise their desire for a child.

This site also provides opportunities to explore adoption of international children. Potential adoptive children from a variety of different countries may be viewed. You may even select criteria and a search will pull up the profiles of the children which may provide the closest match. Your heart will definitely melt after seeing the many children from all parts of the globe, even if you're not seriously exploring international adoption!

Adoption.com also runs articles daily in its Adoption Daily News. Loads of other articles related to adoption may also be found in their Library, which also has a search function to find specific articles.

Easy-to-use live Chat rooms and bulletin boards are also available on the site. And, as if that were not enough, a mall exists where you may purchase additional books, videos, and other goodies.

Adopt: Assistance Information & Support

(http://www.adopting.org)

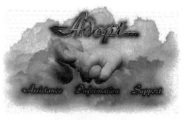

You probably know that Dave Thomas, founder of Wendy's Restaurant, is adopted. But did you know Melissa Gilbert was? And Ted Danson? And Marilyn Monroe? No, this is not what this site is primarily about. But it contains so much information on adoption that there even is an article on <u>Famous Adoptees and Adoptive Parents</u> under their <u>Especially for Adoptees</u> link.

Founded by Sandra Lenington in 1995 Adopt:AI&S strives to be your one-stop adoption source — and it comes very close to doing that! This Web site is so packed full of information, it's a "don't miss" site, even if adoption may still be far from your mind at this point.

If you are just in the process of investigating adoption, make sure to visit the many articles under their <u>Infertility</u> link. Some of my personal favorites include <u>All Things Are Possible</u> and <u>Infertility: School for Parenting</u> (an especially cute article — for it points out how something good can come out of the experience). Be sure to participate in their <u>Support Forums</u> with panel experts such as Patricia Johnston and Graham Wright.

The mystery of <u>The Home Study</u> is finally unraveled in an excellent summary under their <u>FAQs About Adoption</u> link. Want to learn about the various adoption options? Then don't miss information on <u>independent/private, agency,</u> or <u>international adoption</u>. Numerous links to the respective on-line agencies are available under each option. Also be sure to check out their other two sites: http://www.adoption-assist.com and http://www.adopt-usa.com which both contain more information on agencies, and attorneys throughout the USA. The former site also contains a state-by-state guide to waiting children available for adoption.

For those moving into adoption, make sure not to miss Birthmother letters and Enduring the Wait until you Adopt. If you have recently adopted there is much advice regarding Talking to Your Children about Adoption and How do I answer those "rude/awkward" questions people ask me about my children? These and many, many more wonderful articles may be found in their Reading Room, and throughout Adopt: AI&S— so be sure to peruse the whole site thoroughly!

AdoptioNetwork™

(http://www.adoption.org)

Are you seeing a pattern here with the URL addresses? Yes, they can be confusing, but all are different and are wonderful resources to visit.. Started in 1994 by Philip Schulte and Christopher Moore, AdoptioNetwork™ was formed to disseminate information to all parties involved in the adoption process.

This site is much more complex than the others and holds worlds of information as well. Sections are partitioned as they relate to Birthparents, Adoptees, and Parents. AdoptioNetwork™ has a huge listing of agencies (both domestic and international) which are neatly catagorized each by locale. You will also find some invaluable information on laws that govern adoption under Federal Programs. Some Additional Sources offer links to other appropriate articles and sources of information related to adoption.

Adoptive Families of America

(http://www.adoptivefam.org)

Founded in 1966, Adoptive Families of America (AFA) is the largest non-profit organization in the United States to aid adoptive families with information and support. They also support some children who are waiting to be adopted.

AFA publishes the magazine Adoptive Family which is available for purchase on their Web Site. Their Online Catalog also contains a plethora of adoption books, videos, audiocassettes and teaching tools. Their WWW Resources contain many unique links to other sites and mailing lists, some which are as specific as race and nationality, so be sure not to miss this.

adopting.com : Internet Adoption Resources

(http://www.adopting.com)

adopting.com

Welcome to adopting.com - Internet Adoption Resources!

"The largest adoption resources index on the internet"

Here you will find everything prospective adoptive parents need to know about adopting:

- How to get started
- Links to hundreds of adopting agencies, facilitators and attorneys
- Letters to birthparents from families looking to adopt a newborn
- Support groups
- Information on adoptees' rights, perspectives and more
- Emailing lists, newsgroups, bulletin boards and chat
- Waiting child photolistings

Everything you need to know to help you choose the path to adopting that's right for you can be found on the internet, and if it's out there, it can be accessed from adopting.com.

(Disclaimer: Inclusion in this listing does not imply an endorsement of that organization or individual by adopting.com.)

Following in the same light as the previous two sites, adopting.com (different from Adoption.com and, no, it's *not* capitalized) was created by Julie Valentine, an adoptive single mother herself. She is also the Program Coordinator for African Cradle, Inc. (http://www.adopting.com/aci) through which she adopted her daughter, Madison, from Ethiopia. As if all that wasn't enough, she also is the listowner of two mailing groups — XCultureAdopt (cross cultural adoptions) and Single-aparents (single parents adoptions), both of which are easily accessible through this site.

Julie has laid out a very organized beautiful home page. It easily categorizes the different aspects of adoption by hyperlinks to its own subpages or other pertinent sites. As with some of the adoption sites, adopting.com has a section on Getting Started. Letters to Birthparents is also laid out in a unique format for it uses direct links to personal Web pages of those wishing to adopt. You can have your own site added for free. If you are interested and don't have a Web page, Julie also offers design services for those pursuing adoption at reasonable rates.

This site also has information on Agencies, Facilitators, Attorneys, Photolistings which is alphabetized and contains so many links to on-line sources it's amazing. I would highly recommend that if you are searching for an agency in your state to begin your search under this category. Her International Adoption Information and Support by Country sections are also broad and cover over a dozen countries.

National Adoption Information Clearinghouse

(http://www.calib.com/naic/)

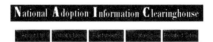

National Adoption Information Clearinghouse

About Us   What's New   Factsheets   Catalogs   Related Sites

The National Adoption Information Clearinghouse (NAIC) was established by Congress to provide professionals and the general public with easily accessible information on all aspects of adoption, including infant and intercountry adoption and the adoption of children with special needs. NAIC maintains an adoption literature database, a database of adoption experts, listings of adoption agencies, crisis pregnancy centers, and other adoption- related services, and excerpts of State and Federal laws on adoption.

NAIC does not place children for adoption or provide counseling. It does however, make referrals for such services.

NAIC is a service of the **Children's Bureau, Administration for Children and Families, U.S. Department of Health and Human Services**.

For more information, contact the National Adoption Information Clearinghouse at:

P.O. Box 1182
Washington, DC 20013-1182
(703) 352-3488
(888) 251-0075
Fax (703) 385-3206
E-mail: naic@calib.com .

Updated on May 29, 1997, by webmaster@calib.com

The National Adoption Information Clearinghouse (NAIC) was established by Congress in 1987 to provide professionals and the general public with easily accessible information on all aspects of adoption, including infant adoption and international adoption, and the adoption of children with special needs. NAIC maintains an adoption literature database; a database of adoption experts; listings of adoption agencies, crisis pregnancy centers, adoptive parent support groups and search support groups; excerpts and full texts of State and Federal laws on adoption; and other adoption-related services and publications. NAIC does not place children for adoption or provide counseling. It does however, make referrals for such services. NAIC is a service of the Children's Bureau, Administration for Children and Families, U.S. Department of Health and Human Services.

Adoption Online Connection®

(http://www.adoptiononline.com)

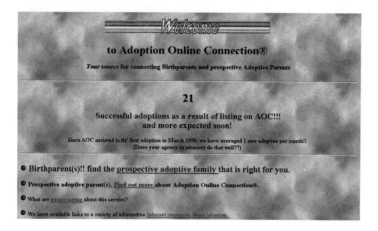

If your are in the process of trying to locate a child, then definitely check out Adoption Online Connection®. Founded by Allison and Charles Chidekel, this service claims to be the first on-line adoption service providing a unique forum to exchange information between birthparents and adoptive parents. Fees are associated with placing information for adoptive parents, but when you consider the audience you are hitting with the Internet this may not be a bad investment. As an adoptive parent, you purchase your own Web page. Birthparents may then view these potential adoptive parents and even search through them based on religion, occupation, residency, marital status or one of the other many preference options.

Rainbowkids.com

(http://www.rainbowkids.com)

Rainbowkids.com is an online international monthly adoption magazine. The founder of the site, Martha Osborne (an adoptive mother herself), wanted to create a Web site and business which gave comprehensive information to those wishing to pursue international adoptions. Rainbowkids.com is not an agency but, like some magazines, it is a company which relies on the advertising of adoption agencies and other related products to provide the information laid out in its Web pages. And, like a regular magazine, each month a cover story is featured, with other articles in the Features section. Some regular information is always included such as International Adoption FAQ, Waiting Children of the World (a Photolisting of Available Children), and Personal Adoption Stories. You can even send a RainbowGram (an e-mail card) on the site to someone who's in the process of adopting. Some other unique features of this site include a Currency Exchange Rate and World Weather for traveling abroad.

FOSTER PARENTING

This book was almost finished when we did our first bit of foster parenting and then I realized that I had almost left an important section out of the book. Foster parenting plays a dual role for the parents and special needs children it serves. The perception of special needs children is often misunderstood. Most of the children in foster homes are not the orphans of long ago nor are they mostly physically handicapped. No, these children have been more permanently scarred in more gruesome ways by physical and sexual abuse. Because of this, they bring with them additional needs which well adjusted children do not require. Many disorders often occur as the result of this abuse and special training is often given to foster and potential adoptive parents of these children.

Becoming a foster parent not only gives you the opportunity to provide a safe temporary environment for special needs children until they are returned home or are placed for adoption, but it also opens a door of opportunity to look at other parenting options. We are so glad we took the opportunity to become foster parents, and I hope that you will use these resources to investigate this option as well.

Foster Parents CARE

(http:// fostercare.org)

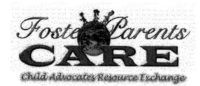

Foster Parents CARE is a non-profit organization dedicated to promoting the safety, enrichment and success of *all* children worldwide. Foster children and adoptive children have a special place in our hearts and our goal is to provide as much information and assistance as possible to help children and their guardians locate the resources they need to ensure every child's success.

We are dedicated to foster and adoptive children and those involved in their care. It is our hope that we can create a true resource on the Internet for all of those involved in the care of foster children. This site is run completely through volunteer efforts. If anyone is interested in helping maintain an area, or has resources that may benefit the children in our care, please contact us. Working together, we can truly make a difference and create a valuable resource.

Foster Parents CARE is still a new site, and is not yet complete, or as comprehensive as we hope it will become

Foster Parents CARE (Child Advocate Resource Exchange) was a nonprofit organization founded to serve the Internet community and dedicated to sharing fostering information. This site contains literally hundreds of links to resources which will help those who are fostering or have been fostered. For foster parents, there are many Foster Parent Links and loads of chat sites, mailing lists, and newsgroups you can join under the Foster Parent Talkabout link. You can even search for previous foster parents, siblings, and children under the Foster Care Search Area. Many recommended books are listed in their Library.

Special Kids :) Special People

(http://www.geocities.com/Heartland/2085/home.html)

This is a very special page indeed, and one of the many links found under Foster Parents CARE. After my short experience with foster children, I about broke down in tears when I came upon this site. Randy and Tina Yows have beautifully designed this page to share some important resources, as well as their experiences with others. If you go to the bottom of this page and double click the MIDI sequence you can peruse the Links For Foster Care or Special Needs Resources, while listening to Phil Collins' *Against All Odds* playing in the background of the site. Tina has also started collecting and writing numerous Poems & Prose which capture the trials and tribuations of caring for special needs children.

CHILDFREE LIVING

In the infertile world this is often spoke of as the "unmentionable option." However, to those who choose this option, the decision of not having children and enjoying *each other as a family* carries with it much relief and a new mindset. No, this in not how it has to end for anyone experiencing infertility, but it is a choice. And couples who choose it often declare how exhilarating it can be, after years of struggling with infertility.

I must confess, coping with this as long as we have, that as time has gone on even my husband and I have considered just going childfree. After our marriage took such a rocky turn a few years back, it made me realize (after we had pulled it out of the gutter) how wonderful just being together is. And that we had so much to be thankful for — just with each other. I can also remember, however, being that new patient just entering treatment shuddering at the thought of childfree living. Because of this change of heart I have come to see the option for what it really is — and have therefore included it so that it is not overlooked. Do yourself a favor and at least investigate the idea — it is an *option*.

A final note of warning, however. Some of these organizations contain both infertile and fertile couples who have chosen not to have children. For some of the fertile couples, population growth control is their reason for going childfree. So, just be prepared for the diverse opinions expressed on these sites.

Childless by Choice

(http://now2000.com/cbc/)

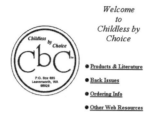

Childless by Choice (CBC) is a good starting point to investigate the option of childfree living. CBC understands the many reasons people choose to be childfree, and therefore they have tried to offer a broad range of information. Originally started as an organization, the husband/wife founding team of this site, consisting of Carin Smith and Jay Bender, has made the site more into a business now. Much valuable information regarding facts, stories, and even humor are available for purchase — at very reasonable prices. They even offer "Still Deciding" packages for couples investigating this lifestyle option. Other products are available which also promote childfree living such as mugs and bumper stickers. Their four years of past newsletters are also available for purchase.

Childfree Resource Network

(http://www.compassnet.com/dmoore/crn/)

This site is fairly well organized and gives much information regarding the childfree lifestyle. However, members of this organization tend to be people who have not experienced infertility. You will still find valuable resources such as Facts and Figures on childfree living and Odd Questions Childfree People are Asked. Have you checked the Resource Page? It is a good collection of books, articles, and other resources on the Childfree lifestyle.

CHAPTER 11

FERTILITY RELATED RESOURCES — BOOKS, PRODUCTS, & SERVICES

Even with all the support in the world, sometimes you just need some added tools to help you in your quest for a child. More and more fertility-related products and services are popping up on the Internet each day. Sad to say, there is a market here — maybe someday there won't be — we can only hope. Anyhow, this chapter is a potpourri of fertility related sites which you may want to investigate.

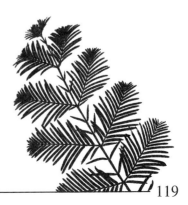

MediNet

(http://www.askmedi.com)

Some of the previously mentioned organizations offer physician referral services which you may want to use. However, if you're really curious about that doctor you are thinking of seeing, or are not pleased with your current one and want to investigate his credentials, then MediNet is the place to go. This reasonably priced service (currently $15 for one doctor, additional docs at $5 up to a maximum of 5 inquires) could save you tremendous future money, time, and headaches. Just some of the information you will find in a MediNet report include:

➡ Medical School and year of graduation

➡ American Board of Medical Specialty Certifications (especially important in identifying Fertility Specialists)

➡ Records of sanctions or disciplinary actions taken against a physician, if any, from all states

and much more.

Adoption Made Easy

(http://www.netxpress.com/users/adoptez/)

If you've ever read *Taking Charge of Infertility* by Patricia Johnston then you'll remember how she repeatedly suggests to persons experiencing infertility to "get a plan." Sometimes it does help a couple to put down in writing what steps will be taken to correct a situation. But how do you know all the options and how to go through the plan in the least amount of time and cost? That's what gave Betsy and David Levin, the founders of this company, the idea that there was a definite need for a service such as this.

Adoption Made Easy can put together a fertility, surrogacy, international or agency adoption plan for you. They are not an agency nor do they give legal or medical advice, but their service may help you same time, money, and valuable emotional resources.

Infertility Counseling Associates

(http://www.mindspring.com/~yepstein/)

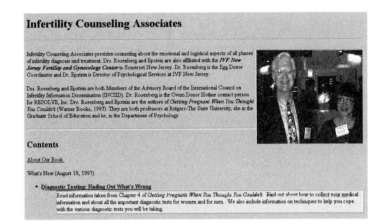

Doctors Epstein and Rosenberg, authors of *Getting Pregnant When You Thought You Couldn't* have developed a Web site and business worth investigating. Although this Web site is constructed to promote their counseling services, loads of other information are abundant on it. Don't miss checking out the list of Activities from their book. From this link you will find valuable infomation such as About 's Infertility, a letter to friends and family on the facts of infertility. There are also exercises on Breathing Relaxation and Mental Rehearsal for Tests/Treatment. And, if you have already enlisted a third-party reproduction assistant, don't miss the Retorts for Third Party Pregnancy.

Tapestry Books

(http://www.tapestrybooks.com)

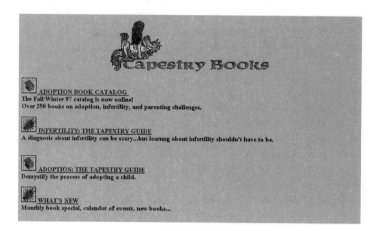

In all of your Web walking you may have stumbled across a title of a book that you would like to purchase. If your local bookstore or library does not carry it, why not check out Tapestry Books? Tapestry Books specializes in carrying a large line of infertility, adoption, and parenting books in their <u>Adoption Book Catalog.</u> Started in 1990 by Laurie Wallmark, Tapestry Books has blossomed from a once mail-order only catalog to this large online source for information. Books for purchase are categorized by subject for easy viewing. Hyperlinks transport you to not only <u>Infertility,</u> but also to <u>Adoption</u> and <u>Parenting Resources</u> as well.

Amazon.com

(http://www.amazon.com)

Amazon.com claims to be Earth's largest bookstore, and after visiting this site myself, I have to admit that it probably is. Aside from their massive collective of all types of books, a major reason for visiting Amazon.com is that they frequently run sales as much as 40% off on featured books. Another nice feature of the bookstore is that you can <u>search</u> by <u>author, title, subject,</u> or even <u>keyword</u> for a book. (When I input the keyword "infertility," Amazon.com pulled up over 200 titles!) They also often carry hard-to-find, or out-of-print books that you can't find anywhere else.

My Forever Family®

(http://www.songnet.com/myforeverfamily/)

Written and Produced by Lisa Silver, a Nashville songwriter and musician, this page mainly was created to promote her album My Forever Family®. The album is about adopting and being adopted and features songs from the anticipation and frustration stages of adoption to the wonderful feelings of bringing the child home. Also included on this page is a Chat site and more Links to other adoption sites. Be warned, however, that currently this page only can be viewed with frames-capable browsers — so if you get an error message that the site cannot be retrieved it is probably because the browser you are using does not support frames.

The Miracle of Adoption: Cards & Announcements

(http://www.adopting.org/cards.html)

This online store specializes in cards, posters, and other adoption-related merchandise. There are Cards for Birthparents, Adoption Announcements, or Cards for those still waiting to Adopt. You may also purchase selected Prints which capture the beauty of adoption, or help promote adoption by purchasing one of their tees or sweatshirts

Custom Adoption Announcements

(http://www.iwaynet.net/~geiger/announce.html)

Another store specializing in unique cards is Custom Adoption Announcements. You may choose from invitations announcing your child's arrival from here or abroad. The adoption announcements are customized to fit whether your new arrival is an infant or young child and include a color picture of your child.

Infertility & Adoption

(http://www.cybertours.com/~msw/)

Infertility & Adoption

Information, guidance, and support for those touched by infertility and/or adoption

Infertility and adoption, both singly and together, are deeply personal and life-altering experiences. They change the way we look at the world. They challenge things we take for granted. They can bring heartache, they can bring great joy.

Infertility is very much like being in a maze. You never know where, or *if*, a solution lies. It's impossible to tell what the ramifications of any choice are: if you pursue conception via one method, does it exclude another method or ruin your chances for still another? Modern medicine presents us with never-ending options, all with great promise, but none with guarantees. We structure our lives around doctor's appointments, wanting to believe that success is imminent. We reach out for miracles, hoping that this month will be different. Some of us are lucky, and the child of our dreams comes to us through biology coupled with persistence, hard work, and luck. For others, our equally magical and perfect children come to us through the gift of adoption. Still others, unable to conceive and not ready to adopt, remain childless.

However our struggle to become parents ends, we are forever changed, as are our relationships with the people around us. An intensely private part of our lives is exposed to the evaluation and scrutiny of others. The validity and wisdom of our decisions are debated. People who mean to be helpful offer unsolicited advice and guidance about something they do not understand. Our spirits are buffeted by the waves of alternating hope and despair.

It become crucial to find people who can listen without judging, people who have gut-level familiarity with what we are going through, people who can witness our struggle no matter how difficult that may be. We at *Infertility & Adoption* have experienced infertility. While we eventually chose adoption, we understand that not everyone does. We feel strongly that your choices, whatever they are, should be honored and respected. We reach out to you with non-judgmental support, accurate information, and knowledgeable guidance.

Infertility & Adoption is also a valuable source of information about adoption, whether or not you come to that choice through infertility. Adoption is a life-long journey, affecting birthparent, adoptive parent, and adoptee. Adoption issues come up at all stages of triad members' lives. We at *Infertility & Adoption* have the experience to help you find a way to deal with adoption issues that's right for you

Infertility & Adoption is a publication of Infertility & Adoption Network in Raymond, Maine. Published six times a year, it primarily focuses on helping people who have experienced infertility and who are contemplating or have chosen adoption. Current subscription rates are $12.95/year.

Roots & Wings Magazine

(http://www.adopting.org/rw.html)

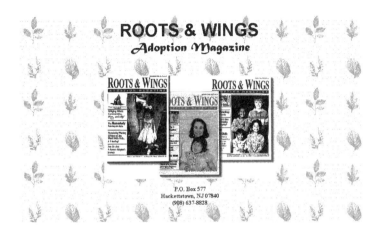

Roots & Wings is a quarterly magazine which covers all aspects of adoption. It exchanges information regarding all aspects of the adoption experience. Many of the articles in the magazine are written by adoptive parents themselves. Some stories a typical issue might include A Baby: From Infertility to Adoption, Building Bridges to your Child's Ethnic Community, and To Tell or Not to Tell (the child's school regarding his/her adoption). Many more articles can be browsed under the Sample Stories section on their home page. Contents of the Current Issue may also be viewed on their page. You can even try your hand at writing by submitting an article under their Sound Off link. Each quarter there is a Feedback Forum where you can add your two cents' worth on a topic which is discussed. The cost of a subscription is currently $19.95/year.

How To Have A Baby
(When the Birds & Bees Let You Down)

(http://www.mindspring.com/~pkwyfert/)

How to Have a Baby was compiled by Beverly Sherrid, a woman who personally fought infertility for seven years and who understands first hand what a couple *really* needs to do if they are having difficulties conceiving. Her book is different in that you may order individual chapters of it online, and her forté in writing it is her ability to convey very technical medical information in layman's terms. A detailed <u>Table of Contents</u> as well as an extensive excerpt of one of the chapters is available to read at this site.

Personal Fertility Tester and
Reproductive Health System

(http://www.pft123.com)

One of the newest ways to track your fertility signs is by observing changes in your saliva. Much like your cervical fluid, saliva also tends to exhibit a "ferning" pattern when viewed under a microscope around fertile times of the month. Although relatively simple in design, most of these devices are quite expensive (currently greater than $50), but the selling point is the easy of use of their products.

Manufactured in California, this saliva reading product was developed by Chain Reactions, Inc. Further information on the company can be found on their home page. A portion of the sales of this product reportedly goes to research of women's fertility programs

DONNA® Fertility Tester

(http://www.jepa.co.uk/berthsol/fertilit.html)

Marketed in the United Kingdom and elsewhere, this saliva reader was developed by BELDAMIO in Rome, Italy. This site also provides information on the clinical tests conducted using the device under <u>Scientific Abstracts.</u>

Lady Free Biotester™

(http://adarweb.com/usbio/)

Manufactured in France, this saliva reader was developed by GTIE Laboratories. In addition, this Web site contains some articles about ovulation and comparison of its product to ovulation predictor kits.

Fertility Forecaster®

(http://www.mpsinc.com/indexfrt.html)

These last two products use computer software for those high-tech fertility buffs, to detect fertile times. Developed by Micro-Processor Systems, Inc. in New York, this software program apparently can predict your fertile periods based on BBT data alone. It claims to use a special algorithm which can predict an upcoming fertile period, based on past data. A research report, demonstration program, and company information is available on their home page.

Conceive Fertility Planner™

(http://www.wie.com/cfp/)

Conceive Fertility Planner was developed by a couple who had themselves experienced problems with fertility. It uses a computer system to track the three common fertility signs — temperature, cervical fluid, and cervical position. The program then automatically draws a cover line and indicates your most fertile times based on your input data. An On-line demo is available to view on the site.

CHAPTER 12

SUCCESS! SUCCESS! OH NO! — MAYBE *TOO MUCH* SUCCESS!

Welcome back to "Colette's Roller Coaster Ride of Infertility"

If any of you have been following my story, I have gotten pregnant through IVF. It was a miracle because it was through a second day ICSI. The first day, my eggs did not fertilize. The clinic I am going to has never had a pregnancy with the second day ICSI.

Well, all along, we have suspected that I might have twins because my pg hormone level has been double of what it should have been. Yesterday, we went for my first ultrasound and saw THREE beating hearts!!! My mouth is still hanging open.

Now we are faced with a huge dilemma. Everyone is talking about Selective Reduction. Before we even attempted IVF, our RE told us of the extremely small chance of triplets and that if it should happen, they suggest that we terminate one. So, we said, "No problem." Now that we have seen those little beating heats, it's a different story. We don't know what to do. I am being released by my RE in two weeks and will have to see a neonatal specialist. That is where we will get our facts to make a decision. On top of all this, I was offered a huge promotion at work yesterday! Can things get any more difficult?

—From the infertility mailing list

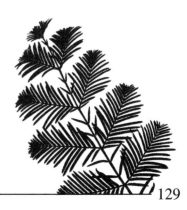

129

This posting captures all too well the other side of the infertility experience. We all so desperately want that longed-for pregnancy, but the upside of success with fertility treatment often results in multiple pregnancies and births. In fact, due to the use of potent fertility drugs and IVF, multiples are now at an all-time high. And, although this sounds like an end to the infertility war and the beginning of an "instant family," multiple pregnancies carry with them a whole other bag of worries, complications, and, sometimes, disappointments. Although most women do not have many problems carrying twins, multiple pregnancies beyond this are often risky to the mother and babies alike. Premature birth is almost always the case in multiples. These early births likewise sometime cause negative health conditions. And the unthinkable — death of the precious babies we've tried so hard to attain and bring into this world — is unfortunately an increased risk associated with carrying and giving birth to multiples.

Because pregnancies and birth of multiples is such a challenging situation, this chapter focuses on several pregnancy and multiples Web sites. Some of these have been developed to specifically deal with the delicate months of carrying multiple pregnancies and coping with the little bundles of joy in the many years to come. I have also included a couple of good all-around pregnancy sites for our wishing pleasure.

ParentsPlace.com

(http://www.parentsplace.com)

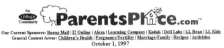

Our Current Sponsors: Bonus Mail | E! Online | Alexa | Learning Company | Kodak | Dell Labs | LL Bean | LL Kids
General Content Areas: Children's Health | Pregnancy/Fertility | Marriage/Family | Recipes | Activities
October 1, 1997

Today's Feature Articles

THIS WEEK: Is Your Computer Hazardous to Your Health? and Parenting News Summary

DENTIST:
Bad Breath in 6.5 Yr Old

KIDS' HEALTH
How to Interpret Oral, Rectal, and Underarm Temperatures

PRESCHOOL:
Getting 3.5 Yr Old to Give Up Pacifier

FAMILY:
My Husband Challenges My Authority in Front of Our Daughter

Bulletin Boards

Index to All Boards

New Boards:
Romance in Marriage?
Single Parents/Dating
Co-Parenting
Noncustodial Parents
Food Issues
Spouse Travels Alot

What's Happening in Our Community Today

SPECIAL CHATS
*April '98 Expecting Club, 12amEDT
*Parents of Teens, 12amEDT
*Christian Parenting, 12amEDT
*Attachment Parenting, 12amEDT
*Breakfast Club Chat, 6amEDT
*Parents Who Work Outside the Home,

You don't need to be a parent yet to visit ParentsPlace.com. This is an extraordinary site with so much information on parenting it will make your head spin. The home page contains featured articles on all aspects of parenting and a listing of chats which change daily. These chats (which are over a dozen topics a day) include subjects such as Infertility, Secondary Infertility, Raising Twins and Multiples, Parents of Preemies and many, many more. Be sure not to miss the READING ROOMS also. Here you will find articles and magazines for Parenting Multiples, Adoptive Parents, and Parenting Special Needs Kids. There also is a place in the reading room to ask questions from professionals such as Midwifes, Doctors, Dentists, Nutritionists, and Preschool Teachers, just to name a few.

Back on the home page you can transport yourself to the Index to all Boards and find a regular Potpourri of topics on the preparation for and the handling of children. Each topic includes a respective tiered bulletin board and these are much nicer than a typical bulletin board or newsgroup. Since the boards are set up in a tiered format it's easy to see responses to each particular question asked.

For those still wishing for that little one there is the Trying to Conceive, Infertility, and the Secondary Infertility bulletin boards along with other topics listed under Pregnancy. Boards under *Family Size* include Twins, Triplets or Higher, and The Only Child. Under the subject of *Family Structure* you will find boards on Adopting Parents, Foster Parents, and Multi-Cultural Families. Many other boards are listed under such topics as *Medical Concerns*, *Losses* (including boards such as Miscarriage and Stillborn), Learning, and *Ages & Stages* (which includes a board on Preemies.)

Stork Site

(http://www.storksite.com)

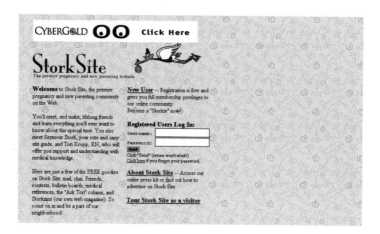

The Stork Site is a fun place to visit. Delightful graphics and a continuously maintained site are some of the secrets which makes this a site one that you will want to return to time and time again, once that little one is on the way. Although you can view a sample of the site as a visitor, to take advantage of the many resources offered by Stork Site you must register as a New User.

Inside this site you will find Storkzine — a constantly updated magazine on parenting including daily articles and news updates. In the Library, you will find a Medical Reference covering topics including High Risk Pregnancy, Maternal Age over 35, Multiple Gestation, and Weight Gain in Pregnancy, in addition to many others. And, if you are still daydreaming of that little one's name, then the Library contains a fun link to The Name Nest. Here you will find thousands of baby names with their meanings and origins. Before leaving their library, check out the Glossary of medical terms, as well as any of the many archived topics.

The Stork Site, of course, has it's own Chat site — The Picket Fence, where you can meet other respective parents or parents-to-be.

Lynne's Ultimate Pregnancy Page

(http://www.geocities.com/Heartland/5552/)

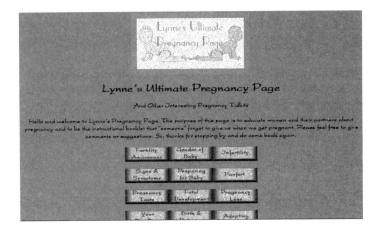

his attractive and well-organized site is the product of a young women named Lynne. An aspiring midwife and computer wiz, Lynne has put together a Web page which covers the whole gambit of motherhood, from <u>Fertility Awareness</u> to <u>Adoption</u>. Much of the information on her pages is original and worth visiting. Feel pregnant? Then check out her information on <u>Signs & Symptoms</u> of pregnancy and <u>HCG levels in Pregnancy</u>. And if you find out you are, then don't miss your chance to guess whether it's a boy or girl under <u>Gender of Baby</u> or <u>Chinese Gender Prediction Chart</u>. And follow the baby's progress under the link to <u>Fetal Development</u>. And for those of us who are *still* trying, check out her <u>Infertility</u> links.

Olen Pregnancy Calendar

(http://www.olen.com/baby/)

When a woman finds out she's pregnant, one of the first things she tries to do is figure out when the baby is due. Now you can do that in a flash, even without a visit to the doctor or trying to count the weeks on a calendar. A visit to this site will allow you to estimate that due date based on the date of your last period or ovulation. Upon entering these dates, the interactive calendar will then calculate not only your due date, but also the week and month in which your pregnancy is now. And for those "planning" to get pregnant, there even is a "what if" ovulation calendar.

The Whole Nine Months

(http://www.homearts.com/depts/health/00ninec1.htm)

This site is easily found when conducting an Internet search dealing with "pregnancy," because it advertises frequently on search engines. In any case, The Whole Nine Months covers more of teh same information as the previous two sites. It, too, contains a pregnancy calendar under When Am I Due? This calendar not only calculates your due date, but also gives your expected baby's horoscope. A variety of pregnancy articles can always be found on the home page. Don't miss How Your Baby Grows, this interactive page describes changes in your baby, your body, and gives advice on prenatal care for each respective month of pregnancy. Be sure to visit Talk to Others and check out the bulletin boards on Women's Health and The Women's Room.

Twins Magazine

(http://www.twinsmagazine.com)

Although titled Twins Magazine, TM is the "magazine for parents of multiples," which sometimes means more than two. This bimonthly magazine can be ordered online by visiting their Subscription and Book Ordering Forms link (currently a subscription runs $23.95/yr US). Other books dealing with multiples can also be found and ordered on this page. Don't know if you want a subscription yet? Then check out some of their Selected Articles which have been put online to view on their home page. Also, their present Table of Contents can always be viewed for each magazine online. Twins Magazine may just be the tool you need to help you deal with your pregnancy and the many challenging years afterward parenting multiples.

Twin Kids

(http://www.hq.net/twinkids/serv.html)

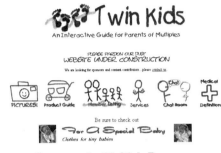

Resources for Multiple Pregnancy

You can help these organizations by passing information on about your multiples.

Center for the Study of Multiple Birth
333 E. Superior St., Suite 476
Chicago, IL 60611

Although still in its infancy (no pun intended), this site contains some valuable resources and will continue to grow through time. John Galbrath, a father himself of twin girls born three months premature, created this site to share what he had learned through his own experience. Twin Kids' <u>Product Guide</u> contains valuable information on where to find strollers and other products for multiples. Their <u>Services</u> include a directory of organizations interested in helping parents of multiples. And, if you are still in the process of carrying the wonderful bundles of joy, you won't want to miss their <u>Medical Definition</u> link. A <u>Chat Room</u> also exists to share stories with others, however, it requires Java software.

Parents of Twins/Multiples

(http://www.lnd.com/twins)

Parents of Twins/Multiples is both a delightful and necessary site to visit if you are expecting more than one. Started as a compilation of information of the <u>Twins/Multiples Mailing List</u> (which you can easily join from their home page) the site continues to grow with information daily. A MUST visit should be their <u>FAQ's</u> link. Here, the author of the site has neatly categorized information from the mailing list into articles on topics including <u>Bedrest with Multiples</u>, <u>Air Travel</u>, <u>Multiples after Infertility</u>, <u>Freebies and Discounts,</u> and dozens more. In addition to the mailing list, a bulletin board is also provided to share additional information and stories.

The Triplet Connection

(http://www.inreach.com/triplets/index.shtml)

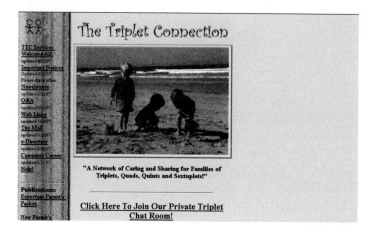

"A Network of Caring and Sharing for Families of Triplets, Quads, Quints and Sextuplets!"

Click Here To Join Our Private Triplet Chat Room!

Although I'm still not expecting, the Triplet Connection is one of my favorite fantasy sites to visit. Created and run by Janet Bleyl (its president and a fellow mother of multiples), this nonprofit organization is dedicated to helping families of triplets or higher multiple births. TTC has a large Scientific Advisory Board comprised of medical experts which you will find information under the TTC Services. TTC's Services also include an Expectant Parent Package, New Parent's Package, and Newsletter. They also offer a Tender Heart's Package for families which have experienced a loss of one or more of their multiples anywhere along the way.

Back on TTC's home page you will find a great resource under the Q & A link. This Bulletin Board answers questions to some frequently asked topics such as Health Questions and tips for Traveling with Triplets. And of course, what woman would not like to go to The Mall and go shopping? Here you will find an extensive amount of strollers, car seats, preemie clothing, books, and other multiple needs which you can purchase.

CHAPTER 13

INTERNATIONAL INFERTILITY RESOURCES

Before you just skip this chapter, remember the reason why the Internet is such an invaluable tool — because it links the *world* together. Although we in America often think that our research far outweighs the rest of the world, we sometimes get a reality check when a medical breakthrough is made half-way around the globe. As a case in point, just recently there was a new breakthrough in Australia which dramatically improved the odds of IVF procedures. Within days this news was on the Internet being shared with doctors and patients everywhere!

In this chapter I have outlined some of the better international sites and organisations which contain fertility and reproductive information. Be sure to visit these sites, for they contain some invaluable information which you may not be able to find on any other sites listed in this book.

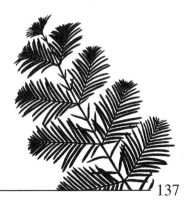

Fertility Awareness & Natural Family Planning

(http://www.fertilityuk.org)

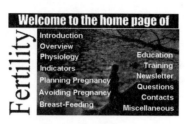

Originating in the United Kingdom, the Fertility Awareness and Natural Family Planning Web site covers the basics of natural family planning and facts about Fertility. Their NFP method is very much like the method taught by Toni Weschler in her book *Taking Charge of Your Fertility*. Although this site may be a bit elementary for those who have battled infertility for a while, it is a good place for starters.

Under the Introduction link you will find both a Fertility Information Quiz and a link to Indicators of fertility. A thorough explanation of how to take, track, and interpret your basal body temperature can be found under this link, as well as how to detect changes in your cervical mucus and position. You may download a copy of their sympto-thermal chart for your use. However, you'll notice that all references to temperatures on it and on this site are in degrees Celsius, rather than Fahrenheit.

Canadian Fertility Resource Site

(http://www.cyberplex.com/CyberPlex/Serono/ferhom.html)

Sponsored by Serono Canada, Inc., this site is a must-visit if you live in Canada. A complete listing of Canadian fertility clinics may be found through a link to their Fertility Centre Directory. You will also find information about Canada's national infertility support network — The Infertility Awareness Association of Canada (IAAC), which has a Bulletin Board link on this Web page. There is also information on how you can get drugs and other procedures covered by your insurance company, along with Sample Drug Benefit Letters to help you do so.

Family Helper

(http://www.helping.com/family/helper.html)

Family Helper came on-line in April 1996 after several years of existing as Toronto Free-Net. And although this Canadian site contains "no fancy graphics, just solid information," it's worth the visit for the valuable services it provides. Family Helper contains an Infertility, Adoption, and Post-adoption section. In fact, the Infertility Helper (featured in Chapter 3) is published by Family Helper and it can be found under the infertility link. In addition to this magazine, they also publish the Adoption Helper and Post-Adoption Helper, available under their respective links.

In the Infertility section you will find links to a number of national and international newsletters, support groups, and fertility clinics. And, whether or not you live in Canada, be sure not to miss the link to the Infertility Network. Much like the IAAC, the Infertility Network offers infertility information and support. On the link to this page, you will find the Articles, Books, Brochures, and Newsletters which they offer. They do accept money orders in US dollars for these items. I recently ordered some articles from them which I received in a timely manner and was pleased that they were very unique and helpful.

Ferti.Net

(http://www.ferti.net)

FertiNet is fully dedicated to the science and practice of Assisted Fertilisation and Human Reproduction. Its primary aim is to stimulate information dissemination among professional workers, researchers and patients in this field.

Public Section
Information on Infertility and Treatment, Patient associations, Fertility centers, Books and more.....

Select your country:

- Australia
- Austria
- Belgium
- Czech Republic
- Denmark
- Egypt
- Emirates
- Finland
- France
- Germany
- Greece
- Hungary
- Iceland
- Israel
- Italy
- Kuwait
- Lebanon
- Netherlands
- Norway
- Poland
- Portugal
- Saudi Arabia
- Spain
- Sweden
- Switzerland
- Turkey
- United Kingdom

Medical Section
ENTER ▶

Monthly updated international magazine, and many features such as information from ESHRE, Human Reproduction, Free MEDLINE, Congress Calendar, Dissertations, Special Interest, Journals, Discussion groups, Case studies and more.

The Medical Section is a **free** service for health professionals only. New visitors are kindly requested to **register** first.

REGISTER ▼

Ferti.Net is the online "Worldwide Fertility Network" and contains a large directory of fertility centers and patient information for over 30 countries and regions in the world. This site, too, is sponsored by Serono. Ferti.Net also has a private communications network for health professions to share reproductive health information.

Under the patient section of the North America link you will find some selected articles under Infertility & Treatment. You may also find more infertility information under other countries, however, most are written in the native language of each country.

International Federation of Fertility Societies (IFFS)

(http://www.mnet.fr/iffs/)

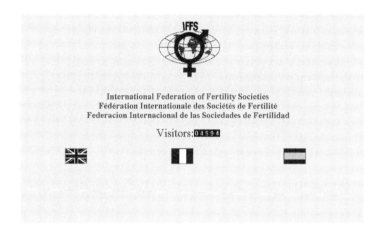

Established over 30 years ago, the International Federation of Fertility Societies (IFFS) is the international organization which binds the world's individual reproductive societies together. They sponsor professional gatherings every three years with members of the world's reproductive societies (the ASRM being America's representative society). The primary goal of the IFFS is to disseminate consistent reproductive health information throughout the world, including countries where established societies do not exist.

Flags of respective countries serve as links to the different language versions of their index. The Union Jack Flag (of the United Kingdom) will take you to their English language version. Under this link you will find more information about the society. A biannual Newsletter and a link to Publications (books, and journals) may be good links to investigate. The Publications section does include links to several online journals — Human Reproduction, Human Reproduction Update, and the Society for the Study of Reproduction. Some of these journals have invaluable articles which you must investigate. Moreover, IFFS releases international consensus data on important questions from time to time. Assisted Procreation Techniques and Tubal Infertility are two such topics and this data will be available in spring of '98.

Society for the Study of Fertility

(http://www.nottingham.ac.uk/ssf/)

The Society for the Study of Fertility is the United Kingdom's equivalent of the American Society for Reproduction Medicine here in the states. Their Web site is well organized and very colorful. However, it currently is entirely geared toward only professionals in the field. They do provide a newsletter, but it is only available in PDF and postscript form. For patients, the main reason it is listed here is because I envision that they may offer patient information in the future (much like the ASRM does now).

Infertility in the United Kingdom

(http://www.bris.ac.uk/Depts/ObsGyn/crm/welcomez.htm)

Infertility in the United Kingdom is cosponsored by the Centre for Reproductive Medicine (in Bristol) and Organon, the other major fertility medication manufacturer. Don't miss this site! It is an excellent one providing Basic Information regarding Infertility. A very helpful book can also be found on this site titled The Infertility Patient Directory. This guide gives you more tips on how to be a successful fertility patient and covers topics including male infertility, secondary infertility, and counseling. The Useful Patient Information provided by Organon includes illustrated articles on:

- Polycystic Ovarian Syndrome

- Male Infertility

- IVF & GIFT

- Ovulation Induction

- Intrauterine Insemination and

- A Global Snapshot of IVF in 1994, which I'm sure will be updated and includes statistics worldwide.

Access

(http://www.ozemail.com.au/~accessoz/)

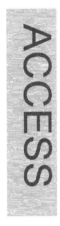

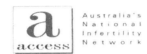

Australia's
National
Infertility
Network

- What is ACCESS?
- Infertility Information
- Fact Sheets
- Australian Infertility Links
- International Infertility Links
- Membership Enquiries
- Contacting ACCESS

You are visitor # 144 since 1st January 1997

This page was created for ACCESS by MS Soft Pty Ltd. If you have any problems viewing this page please email MS Soft. This page was updated on August 14, 1997

Access is Australia's National Infertility Support Network for support and information dissemination. You may want to visit their site to look at the Fact Sheets they have to offer. Like RESOLVE and the Infertility Network, Access charges a minimal fee for these fact sheets, and you must send Australian dollars to order. However, since Australia seems to have a fairly aggressive infertility research program, they might be worth the hassle if you are hungry for information on a specific topic.

European Infertility Network

(http://www.nics.gov.uk/cinni/ein/)

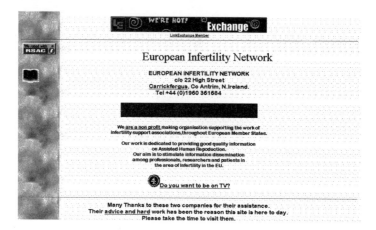

The European Infertility Network is a non-profit organisation which provides information and support the whole European community. This highly animated site offers information on the female and male causes and treatments of infertility. It also contains links to all European countries and other countries around the world for advertisement of clinics, organisations, and other pertinent information. The site also contains links to European journals, societies, and organisations throughout Europe. One of these, ISSUE (The National Fertility Association of the UK), offers support much like RESOLVE does here in the States. Another, the International Federation of Infertility Associations, aims at compiling and sharing infertility information from all associations and organisations throughout the world.

CHAPTER 14
LEARNING HOW TO SEARCH
FOR THE INFO YOU NEED MOST

By the time you've reached this chapter, hopefully you've tried to check out some of the sites listed in this book. But in the course of trying to pull up a particular site, even though you've checked and rechecked all of your spelling, you may have gotten an error message instead of the site. "What has happened?," you ask. The site may or may not still exist, but how do you know? You've now discovered one of the many reasons why it's necessary for you to learn how to search the Internet. But what if all of the site addresses listed in this book are still correct? (A highly unlikely event by the very nature of the ever-changing Internet) Why must you then learn how to search the Internet?

In this chapter we will explore the many reasons why you must learn to search. And as I've already shown you, there are many different systems which run on the Internet. So, in addition to searching Web pages, we will learn how to search newsgroups which often offer some personal accounts and tips of their own. We will also look how to set up new mailing lists. This chapter will be invaluable to you for it will show you how to hunt for and find that particular piece of information which you are seeking. And, through it all, you will also learn how to cut your search times down substantially.

WHY YOU NEED TO LEARN HOW TO SEARCH THE INTERNET

Remember that the biggest selling point regarding the Internet is the fact that it offers the latest *up-to-date* information available anywhere. The Internet is an ever-changing informational source. Because of this, Web sites will change, move, or disappear completely in the course of time while new sites will be added. Constant discussion on Newgroups and mailing lists grows every minute. Let's look at some of the specific instances when you will need to search the Internet:

"I'm getting an error message when I go to call up a Web site."

As previously mentioned, this may be the first reason to prompt you to want to learn how to search. There are several reasons why you might be getting an error message. If the site has not been misspelled, you may be getting an error message due to the fact that the Web page may not be running at that present

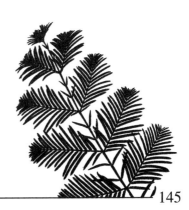

time on its particular server. If you remember from Chapter 1, Web sites must reside on a server (a person's or company's computer) which must be on and looped into the Internet for others to call up and view the site. If the server's computer system is down its resident Web pages will not be viewable. This happens from time to time, especially when the server is conducting maintenance on their computers. Should this be the case, you should be able to pull the site up with that particular address within a day or two.

If you do not wish to wait, of if you have waited and the site still cannot be pulled up, then another reason you may be getting an error message is that the page may no longer be on that particular server at all. Authors of Web pages from time to time move their pages to other servers for whatever reason. In this case, the URL address will have changed. Sometimes, the author of the site may have renamed the URL address completely for ease of remembrance and added marketing to his visitors. Never fear, you can still find this site by learning how to search for it.

"I wonder if there are any new infertility sites?"

New sites = more information. Sometimes they contain just the information which you need most. They might be created by an organization, health professional, individual, or a new clinic close to home which has started advertising on the Web. In any case, we will explore how to make sure you do not miss any of the new sites which come on-line.

"My specialist said that I've been diagnosed with_____ and I want to know more about it"

OR

"I'm going to have a _____ procedure. What can I expect?"

Remember, although I've tried to do a thorough job at outlining the major sites dealing with infertility in this book, the Internet, particularly the Web, is growing at a lightning pace. Information on sites is being updated daily. And, there will be continue to be more sites, I guarantee, on this subject by the time this book goes to press. So if you want to find out options for "unexplained infertility" or about your diagnosis of "premature ovarian failure," you can find out loads of information on very specific topics, once you've mastered the art of searching.

As I've previously mentioned, it is pertinent to cross-reference all that you read on the Internet with reliable sources, either elsewhere on the Net or with your doctor. Searching also allows you to do some cross-referencing on specific topics from different Internet or printed sources.

"I wonder if this information in this book I have (dated _____) is still accurate regarding my condition?"

Although books (especially those written by medical professionals) tend to have invaluable information in them, technology advances are made daily. What a doctor might have claimed in a book even 2-3 years old may now be not completely true. I remember reading a book dated 1987 talking about luteal phase defects. At the time, natural progesterone treatment was just in its infancy and the author of this particular book basically told the reader that luteal phase defect problems still remain elusive. Well, since then, as those of you with this condition well know, natural progesterone treatment works wonderfully in most of these cases for this condition. Granted, most people tend to read up-to-date books, but with the technology growing at lightning speed, why not investigate if new advances have been made on your condition, especially if the pathology is not good? These advances may come from half way around the world, and although your doctor may not appreciate your investigations and inquiry, remember that you are the patient and that it is your money and body. At the very least, doing this may help your decision making and peace of mind in taking such an active role.

SO WHAT ARE THE VARIOUS SEARCH TOOLS AVAILABLE AND HOW DO I USE EACH?

As there are many different systems which run on the Internet, so, too are there different tools to wade through all of that information. You will use different tools to search through newgroups and Web pages.

Web pages

There are millions and millions of Web pages. To sift through all of these Web pages and find information, you will need to use either a "search engine" or "directory." The number of search engines and directories out there are numerous, and all reside on their own Web pages, so no new software is necessary to use them. However, knowing how to make the most of them is the "art" of successful searching. Let's first look at the differences between search engines and directories, then we will get into specifics on how to actually use them.

Search Engines vs. Directories

Many people speak about search engines and directories interchangeably, probably because they look so similar on the surface. In fact, both search engines and directories are located like any other site on the Internet and each has its own address. (For an extended list of search engines and directories check out Appendix C). But each works completely differently from the other.

Search engines use a computer system to wade through all the many millions of pages out on the net. Most search engines are run and operated by different companies, so each search engine's programming varies a bit. Some search engines only search through the titles and summaries of a Web page, while others search the entire text of a document. It is unlikely that you will ever find out exactly how each search engine operates, mainly because the business of search engines is competitive. Every company offering a search engine wants you to use their search engine, so why would they tell anyone just exactly how it operates in fear that others might follow? You can get an idea of how one operates, however, just by the use of it over time.

What we do know about search engines in general (and how they differ from directories) is that they search using a mechanism known as a "spider." (Get it? — Web, spider — cute, huh?) This spider weaves in and out of all of the text contained in the millions of pages which exist on the Web. As the spider weaves in and out of documents, it categorizes words, phrases, or concepts and sorts them into an index. Once again, search engines vary as to how many times a spider passes over every Web page. Some make a pass through all of the Web pages once every 3 days, some only once every week. As you can imagine, the best search engines are the ones that have spiders which crawl through the Web on a more frequent basis, and those that will categorize and index better than others.

Directories, on the other hand, use people to do the searching. The companies which run directories have people who literally spend their days taking sites which are reported to them by the site owners and then neatly categorizing them into indexes. Much like a librarian sorting through and classifying a stack of new books, these services try to categorize Web sites into a logical order. One of the major disadvantages of this service, however, is that Web pages which are not reported to the service are overlooked. Therefore, where a search engine might be scanning millions of Web pages, a directory may only include a fraction of those reviewed Web pages. However, directories tend to be excellent tools if you are searching by subject, since this is how the people behind the scenes typically classify — in neat, categorized order.

Where directories truly fall short is when you are looking for a *relationship* between two different subjects matters. Say you are looking for a relationship, such as between "bacteria" and its causes of "infertility." If you type in "bacterial causes of infertility" in a directory it will more than likely give you search results which shown Web pages discussing only "bacterial cause" not necessarily related to "infertility", or vice versa. Once again, finding a document which contains the effects of bacteria on infertility via a directory is not easy since directories use human topic sorting. Note, however, that it is not necessarily the amount of words in a phrase which will dictate when to use a search engine instead of a directory. You may find information on a three (or more) word phrases such as "human menopausal gonadotropins" via a directory because those three words comprise one general topic or concept which can be neatly categorized.

Some search engines, on the other hand, use a sorting mechanism known as Boolean logic to combine words so that you can find documents which contain both topics that thus may contain the relationship which you are seeking. Once again, as with all search engines, it is hard to tell which ones inherently use Boolean logic, but sometimes these are available, if not obvious, under the "advanced features" section of a particular search engine. Words such as "and," "or," "near," or "not," are what are called Boolean operators. Boolean operators help a search engine weed through and sort out documents which contain one or more of the topics. The way Boolean logic works is illustrated below. Figure 14-1 illustrates an "and" operator. Only documents which contain both subjects will be displayed as findings by the search engine. This document shows the example of "bacterial causes" AND "infertility."

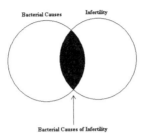

Figure 14-2 shows the combined use of "and" and "not" operators. By combining operators, you can narrow your search even more. This example shows how a search engine would look for "female" AND "infertility" and NOT "hormonal problems."

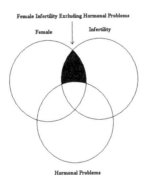

As I mentioned, some search engines will automatically use the "and" operator when two or more words are entered. However, you will likely need to use the advanced features of a search engine to use operators such as "or" , "near," or "not."

The term "NEAR" in some search engines' advanced features is excellent for narrowing a search between an otherwise typical subject that a directory may not have classified. Going back to the previous example, "embryo adoption" is a subject that many directories will not find. Although many search engines will find plenty articles containing the words "embryo" AND "adoption" in them, these may be covering anything from general infertility to abortion. But what you are really looking for is the subject phrase "embryo adoption." By use of the term "NEAR" it tells the search engine only to retrieve those articles where the word "embryo" is very close is proximity in the document to "adoption." You therefore get a much narrower search.

Meta Search Engines

There are also search engines out there which search other search engines' findings. These are called Multiple or Meta Search Engines. They are particularly helpful if you are just starting out a search on a complicated multi-word phrase or trying to find a relationship between several topics. You may want to use a meta search engine *first* when doing this type of search to find which individual search engine is retrieving the best results for that particular query. Then you can refine that search more within that particular search engine. I have found this technique particularly useful.

The dawn of a new service — the Guided Tour

There is a new service which is quickly becoming popular and provides yet another route to find information by category or subject. Much like a directory, guided tours use people to sort, categorize, and rate Web pages based on the particular subject. Some of these companies allow anyone to become a guide for any subject. And, because some of the companies pays their guides to cover a subject area, the subjects are well surfed and intend to be categorized better than a typical directory. At the present time, there are only a couple guided tour companies but I'm sure the idea will catch on and that more of these searching tools will be available in the future. As of this writing, no one had stepped up to the plate to be the guide for an "infertility" subject at the Mining Company (www.miningco.com), but I'm sure that will not remain that way for long. BabyZone[sm] (www.babyzone.com) has several Web pages on Infertility reviewed. Check them out!

So, in summary of this section, use directories when you are looking up specific *subjects*, and search engines when you want to find certain *relationships*. A listing of some of the many search engines and directories can be found in Appendix C. Note that these are just a handful of the hundreds of search tools available. I have also listed some Web pages which keep up and have access to the many search engines available. Overtime you will develop your own likes and dislikes of the various search tools laid out in this Chapter.

Newsgroups

Searching for information in newsgroups is sometimes a lot easier and can uncover some real gems in your results. However, be aware that the information on any given posting is one person's opinion, based on his or her experience, and that that person usually is not a professional in the subject matter. Nevertheless, searching newsgroups gives you the ability to find a person or persons with exactly the same diagnosis, treatment, or situation you are experiencing. You may then e-mail these people directly for additional information and support.

One of the best tools for searching through information on newsgroups is DejaNews which is basically a search engine which leafs through millions of postings dated back to March 1995 for the key words you enter. Here's a tip if you are searching newsgroups for multiple word phrases, however — use the advanced features! As an illustration, type in the phrase "embryo adoption" in the window of the home page of DejaNews. You'll be surprise to find postings pulled up from all kinds of newsgroups such as "alt.abortion," "misc.pregnancy.kids," and "alt.society.liberal." If you look at the contents of these postings, you'll notice that indeed all contain the words "embryo" and "adoption" but not necessarily "embryo adoption." The Power Search ability on DejaNews allows you to easily narrow your search. For instance, if you type in the phrase "embryo adoption" into the Power Search on DejaNews, it will pull up that exact topic in the newsgroups such as "alt.infertility," "alt.adoption," and "alt.adoption.agency."

DejaNews also has the ability to find newsgroups dealing with subject matters. If you type in "infertility" in the window and choose "Find newsgroups," DejaNews will pull up all newsgroups which contain that topic.

Other search engines have the ability to search through newsgroups also, but DejaNews is particularly easy to use and I find it has a nicer format. Check out Appendix C for a listing of other search engines which have a newsgroup searching feature.

MAILING LISTS

E-mail, luckily, is a bit more private. At the present time there is no software which can sift through the enormous amount of personal mail sent electronically — that includes mail sent through mailing lists. However, a number of services can help you set up your own mailing list if you are interested. Sparklist is one of the services which can help you do this and is located at:

www.sparklist.com

Loads of information on the features of mailing lists, how they work, and how to set one up for yourself is discussed in detail on their site.

SOME TIPS ON HOW TO NARROW YOUR SEARCH QUICKLY

Although I have tried to outline the basic tools used for successful searching, there really are no "right" or "wrong" ways of searching the Net. The way you search, however, will cut down the time it takes to find that precious gem you're looking for. Because the tools used to search the Internet are in constant flux, it's hard to outline exactly which specifics each search tool offers. (I have included highlights of some of the search tools in Appendix C, however.) Therefore, I wanted to close this chapter by listing some tips which may aid you in fine tuning your searches.

➡ As previously mentioned, use directories first for *subject* searches, and actual search engines for *relationship* searches. Use Meta search engines to find out which particular search engine is performing best for your specific search.

➡ Use as few words as possible at first, and then build your search by adding one word at a time.

➡ Use the advanced features of a search engine when possible.

➡ Use the most specific terms in your search *first* if you are conducting a relationship search. If you are looking for "infertility caused by bacteria," — it's better to type in "bacterial causes of infertility" since the phrase itself is more specific.

➡ Use unique words, where possible.

If all else fails, you can find more tips and resources for searching at either:

issfw.palomar.edu/Library/TGSEARCH.HTM

or check out Yahoo's *Searching the Web* tips at:

www.yahoo.com/Computers_and_Internet/Internet/World_Wide_Web/ Searching_the_Web.

Enjoy the wonderful resources which the Internet can bring to you and, once again, Happy Surfing!

GLOSSARY OF TERMS

Internet Terms

bits per second (bps): Computer data is comprised of tiny bits of information. Modems vary as to how fast they can transfer this data and this transfer speed is rated in bits-per-second. The current fastest modems transfer data as fast as 56,000 bps.

bulletin board: Similar to bulletin boards used in the tangible world, electronic bulletin boards provide a place on Web sites or other online services to post and read messages.

electronic mail (e-mail): One of the oldest computer systems on the Internet. Similar to real mail in the tangible world, e-mail is an electronic version of mail that can be sent back and forth to other persons and groups. Like an official memo in the business world, messages may be copied to others.

file transfer protocol (FTP): Another older computer system on the Internet allowing users to transfer files between computers. Typically used when transferring Web pages from the Webmaster to the server that holds the Web pages.

gopher: Another original system on the Internet that primarily consisted of files neatly categorized by the use of menus on servers. An analogy may be to envision files filed away into cabinets (the server or gopher). Gopherspace consisted of the ability of interconnection of the gophers. It is possible to search through all gophers by using search tools such as Veronica or Archie.

hardware: A tangible piece of computer equipment. Computer terminals, screens, modems, keyboards, and speakers are examples of hardware.

hotbutton: *see link*

hotlink: *see link*

hyperlink: *see link*

hypertext markup language (HTML): The computer language used to develop Web pages.

hypertext transfer protocol (HTTP): The system used on the Internet which transfers and constructs various graphic, sound, and text files into Web pages.

icon: A picture on a Web page or in a computer program that, when clicked on, causes the program to perform an execution. Within a Web page, icons are used as navigational tools to transfer the viewer to other Web pages.

Internet: The interconnection of and communication between computers through-out the whole world.

Internet service provider (ISP): A company which provides computer hard drive space (where Web pages can reside) and Internet access. ISPs often also provide electronic mail service, file transfer protocol, or any of a number of other computer-related services. Apart from maintenance related downtime, ISP computers run non-stop, allowing constant access to the Web pages that reside on their computers.

ISDN (Integrated Services Digital Network): A much faster digital transmission service (as opposed to normal phone lines) which runs at speeds up to 128 kilobits-per-second.

link: As it relates to the World Wide Web, a tie from one Web page to another Web page. On a Web page, a link typically appears as an icon or an underlined word.

mailing list: A group of people sharing and discussing a common interest. To join the list participants must subscribe to it using a common command via an e-mail message. A computer system distributes messages "posted" by any member of the group to all members of the list via electronic mail.

modem: A piece of computer hardware that uses a phone line to communicate between other computer systems.

newsgroup: Similar to a bulletin board, a place where people sharing a common interest can post and read messages. Unlike bulletin boards, members must first "subscribe" to a newsgroup using a newsreader.

newsreader: A piece of software that allows a person to subscribe, read, and post messages to a newsgroup.

online service company: A company that provides a piece of software which, when loaded on a computer, allows the viewer easy access to the Internet. Besides e-mail, and newsgroup readers, online service companies usually provide additional services beyond that of an Internet service provider.

ram: Also known as computer memory, a capability rating of a computer that holds the currently executable program(s) that are running on the computer systems. Computers with higher ram capacity run more programs at the same time. Some of the current ram capabilities are as high as 128 megabytes.

search engine: A company on the World Wide Web providing a system that searches through various Web pages and retrieves very specific criteria entered by the user of the search engine. Search engines reside on Web pages themselves, and can be accessed simply by entering their specific URL address in a Web browser.

server: A computer system that usually holds Web pages and is used by customers to access many other systems on the Internet.

software: A computer program which can be loaded and run on a computer. Spreadsheets, databases, word processors, and any system that runs on a computer are examples of computer software.

surf: Usually applying to the World Wide Web, moving from one Web page to another, usually in a random fashion. Shopping is a good analogy.

uniform resource locator (URL): The official address of a Web or Gopher page. It is a standardized system used on the Web to find Web sites. URLs are entered in a Web browser to pull up a specific site.

Web browser: A piece of software used to pull up sites and aid in navigation around the Internet. Web browsers currently include Netscape Navigator and Internet Explorer.

Web master: The creator of a given Web site.

World Wide Web (WWW or Web): One of the most popular systems residing on the Internet. The Web uses a system that can compile various graphics, sound, and text files into a page that is visually appealing and interactive.

Fertility Terms

Now you should know by now that *you* need to look these up for yourself! Check out these specific pages:

www.inciid.org/glossary.html

www.fertilitext.org/gloss.htm

www.fertilitycenter.com/definitions.htm

www.reproductivescience.com/glossary.htm

www.ihr.com/ivfphoenix/fertbook/glossary.htm

APPENDIX A

FERTILITY RELATED NEWSGROUPS

alt.infertility .... discussion over whole range of infertility

alt.infertility.primary .... support/discussion of individuals fighting primary infertility

alt.infertility.secondary .... support/discussion of individuals fighting secondary infertility

alt.infertility.pregnancy .... discussion of pregnant individuals who have fought infertility

alt.infertility.alternative .... discussion on alternative medicine and techniques for achieving fertility

misc.health.infertility .... discussion on medical aspects of infertility

alt.support.pco .... support/discussion of individuals diagnosed with PCO

alt.support.des .... support/discussion of individuals who have been affected by DES

soc.support.pregnancy.loss ..... support after pregnancy loss

alt.adoption.agency .... support/discussion on adoption

alt.support.foster-parents .... discussion of experiences of foster parents with special needs children

sci.med.obgyn .... general female medical discussion

APPENDIX B

FERTILITY CLINICS, PHARMACIES, SURROGACY & EGG DONORS,
AND SPERM BANK DIRECTORY

FERTILITY CLINICS

DOMESTIC
ARIZONA

Phoenix

IVF Phoenix
www.ihr.com/ivfphoenix
Arizona Institute of Reproductive
 Medicine, Ltd.
www.conceive.com

Tuscon

University Medical Center - Fertility
 Program
www.ahsc.arizona.edu/~umc/
fertitl.htm

CALIFORNIA

Alamo

Woman to Woman Fertility Center
www.ihr.com/woman/index.html

Beverly Hills

West Cost Infertility & Reproductive
Associates
www.ihr.com/westcoast

Irvine

Werlin Zarutskie Fertility Centers
www.wzfertctr.com

Loma Linda

Loma Linda University Center for
Fertility and In Vitro Fertilization
home.earthlink.net/~lluivf

Laguna Niguel

Werlin Zarutskie Fertility Centers
www.wzfertctr.com

Redondo Beach

Center for Advanced Reproductive
 Care
www.inciid.org/wisot.html

Sacramento

Pacific Fertility Medical Center
www.ns.net/users/doctorg/index.htm

San Diego

IGO Medical Group of San Diego
www.ihr.com/igo
Scripps Clinics
www.scrippsclinic.com/centers/fertil/

San Francisco

University of California, San
Francisco, U.C. Medical Center
Department of Obstetrics,
Gynecology, and Reproductive
Sciences
www.ihr.com/ucsfivf
San Francisco Center for Reproductive
Medicine
sfivf.com
Stanford Health Services
Reproductive Endocrinology and
Infertility Division
www-leland.stanford.edu/dept/
GYNOB/rei

San Ramon

Bay Area Fertility & Gynecology
   Medical Group
Walnut Creek & San Ramon
www.ihr.com/bafertil

Santa Monica

Dr. Richard Marrs
www.inciid.org/marrs.html

Santa Rosa

California North Bay Fertility
   Associates
www.ihr.com/cnbfa

San Jose & Palo Alto

Fertility Physicians of Northern
California
www.ihr.com/fpnc

Portola Valley

Peninsula Fertility - Online
www.conception.com

Southern California

The Fertility Institutes & Southern
   California Surrogate Pregnancy
   Center
www.fertility-docs.com
Scripps Clinic Fertility Center
www.scrippsclinic.com/centers/fertil
Southern California Centers for
   Medicine & Women Care
www.sandiego.sisna.com/minho/
   index.html
West Coast Fertility Centers
www.ivfbaby.com

Redding

The North State Women's Center
www.ihr.com/nswc

COLORADO

Denver

Colorado Reproductive Endocrinology
www-108.rmi.net/crecares.html

Englewood

The Center for Reproductive Medicine
www.falcontech.com/babies

DELAWARE

Newark

Cooper Institute
www.jhcheck.com

FLORIDA

Boca Raton

Fertility Institute of Boca Raton
fertilityboca.com
Boca Raton & West Palm Beach
Palm Beach Fertility Center
www.icapro.com/pbfertil

GEORGIA

Atlanta

Atlanta Reproductive Health Centre
www.ivf.com
Reproductive Biology Associates
www.rba-online.com

Augusta

Augusta Reproductive Biology
   Associates
www.csranet.com/~sknox/arba.htm

HAWAII

Honolulu

Reproductive Innovations
   International
www.surfhi.com/fii/fii.htm

IOWA
Iowa City
UIHC Advanced Reproductive Care
www.uihc.uiowa.edu/pubinfo/arc.htm

ILLINOIS
Chicago
Advanced Fertility Center of Chicago
www.advancefertility.com
Center for Human Reproduction
www.centerforhumanreprod.com
Reproductive Medical Program
  - Dr. Beer
*www.finchcms.edu/clinic/
  beerwww.html*

Oakbrook
Oak Brook Fertility Center
www.inciid.org/oakbrook.html

INDIANA
Merrillville
Center for Human Reproduction
www.centerforhumanreprod.com

Bloomington
Indiana University Fertility Program
*www.medlib.iupui.edu/obgyn/
  infert.html*

IOWA
Iowa City
Assisted Reproductive Technologies
  (ART)
University of Iowa Hospitals and
  Clinics
129.255.16.57/pubinfo/arc.htm

West Des Moines
Mid-Iowa Fertility
www.netins.net/showcase/mifertility

LOUISIANA
New Orleans
The Fertility Institute
www.fertilityinstitute.com

MAINE
South Portland
The Fertility Center of Maine
*www2.coastalwh.com/coastalwh/
  home.html*

MARYLAND
Baltimore
Fertility Center of Maryland
www.erols.com/fcmivf/index.html
The GBMC Fertility Center Baltimore
www.gbmc.org

Gaithersburg
Genetics & IVF Institute
www.givf.com

Rockville
Shady Grove Fertility Center
www2.shadygrovefertility.com/sgfc

MASSACHUSETTS
Boston
Boston Center for Reproductive
  Medicine
members.aol.com/IVFinfo/index.html
Faulkner Centre For Reproductive
  Medicine
www.choicemall.com/ivfinfo

MISSOURI
The Infertility Center of Saint Louis
www.infertile.com

NEW JERSEY

Bayonne

Cooper Institute
www.jhcheck.com
also in **Marlton**

Engelwood

Phillip Lesorgen, MD
www.holyname.org/physpage/
lesorgen.htm

Lawrenceville & Plainsboro

Delaware Valley OB/Gyn and
Infertility Group, PC
www.delvalobgyn.com

New Brunswick

Robert Wood Johnson Medical School
Division of Reproductive
Endocrinology and Infertility
www.rwj-obgyn.umdnj.edu/divisions/
REPROEN/REPRO1.HTM
also in **Princeton**

Somerset

IVF New Jersey Fertility &
Gynecology Center
www.ivfnj.com

West Orange

West Essex Center for Advanced
Reproductive Endocrinology
www.angelfire.com/nj/wecare/
index.html

NEW MEXICO

Albuquerque

Southwest Fertility Services
www.southwestfertility.com

NEW YORK

Brooklyn

Brooklyn IVF
www.brooklyn-ivf.com

Cornell

The Center for Reproductive Medicine
and Infertility
www.inciid.org/rosenwaks.html
Center for Male Reproductive
Medicine and Microsurgery
www.inciid.org/goldstein.html

New York

MacLeod Laboratory
www.fertilitysolution.com
Long Island Fertility & Endocrinology
www.LongIslandIVF.com
The Center for Reproductive Medicine
and Infertility at The New York
Hospital-Cornell Medical Center
www.ivf.org

NORTH CAROLINA

Cary

North Carolina Center for
Reproductive Medicine
www.fuzz.com/nccrm

Chapel Hill

University of North Carolina
www.med.unc.edu/obgyn/infonl/

OHIO

Dayton

Genetics and IVF Institute of Ohio
(GIVF)
www.erinet.com/givf

PENNSYLVANIA

Abington

Abington Reproductive Medicine
www.abington-repromed.com

Danville

Fertility Center at Geisinger Medical
Center
www.hslc.org/~rshabanowitz

Hershey

Reproductive Endocrinology at Penn
State Geisinger, The Milton S.
Hershey MedicalCenter
*www.hmc.psu.edu/depts/obgyn/
repend.htm*

Melrose Park

Cooper Center
www.jhcheck.com

Philadelphia

The Women's Institute of Fertility,
Endocrinology, and Menopause
www.womensinstitute.org
also in **Plymouth** and **Langhorne**

SOUTH CAROLINA

Mt. Pleasant

Southeastern Fertility Center
www.sims.net/soufe

TENNESSEE

Johnson City

Center for Applied Reproductive
Science
www.ivf-et.com

TEXAS

Houston

University of Texas OB/GYN and
Reproductive Sciences
obg.med.uth.tmc.edu/home.html

San Antonio

Fertility Center of San Antonio
www.ihr.com/fcsa

VIRGINIA

Annandale

Shady Grove Fertility Center
www2.shadygrovefertility.com/sgfc

Arlington

Dominion Fertility and Endocrinology
www2.dominionfertility.com/df/
also in **Reston** and **Washington D.C.**

Fairfax

Genetics & IVF Institute
www.givf.com

Norfolk

Jones Institute for Reproductive
Medicine
www.evms.edu/jones/depthome.htm

WASHINGTON

Seattle

The Fertility and Endocrine Center of
the University of Washington
Medical Center
*weber.u.washington.edu/~uwfec/
FEC_Webpages/Index.html*

WISCONSIN

Milwaukee

Reproductive Specialty Center
www.execpc.com/~rsc

Rochester

The Division of Reproductive
  Endocrinology and Infertility at
  Mayo Clinic
www.mayo.edu/repro/re_main.htm

INTERNATIONAL

AUSTRALIA

Perth, WA and Canberra, ACT

Concept Fertility Centre
www.conceptfert.com.au

Queensland

Queensland Fertility Group
www.geocities.com/HotSprings/2952/

Sydney

Sydney IVF
www.sivf.com.au/

CANADA

BRITISH COLUMBIA - Vancouver

Genesis Fertility Centre
www.iatronet.net/genesis
University of British Columbia
www.iatronet.net/ubc-ivf

ONTARIO - Ottawa

Ottawa Civic Hospital
www.conceive.org

ONTARIO - Scarborough

IVF Canada
www.ivfcanada.com

ONTARIO - Toronto

Toronto Centre for Advanced
  Reproductive Technology (TCART)
www.medpathways.com/tcart/

QUÉBEC - Mount-Royal

PROCREA, Fertility Centre
www.infertility.ca

QUÉBEC - Ville Mont-Royal

Procrea Biosciences inc.
www.procrea.ca

DENMARK

Copenhagen

IVF Fertility Clinic The Triangle
home4.inet.tele.dk/fertil/

Frederiksberg

Danish Fertility Clinic
inet.uni-c.dk/~hoest/index.html

NEW ZEALAND

Auckland -Takapuna

North Shore Fertility
*www.hospitals.co.nz/artemis/
  facility1.html*

SWEDEN

Fertility Centre Scandinavia
www.fertilitetscentrum.se

ALSO SEE:

Individual Directories listed on
  Fert.Net
http://ferti.net

ON-LINE PHARMACY DIRECTORY

DOMESTIC

BRAUN FERTILITY
www9.interaccess.com/bdrugs/

DANDURAND DRUGS
www.witchitadirect.com/dandurand

FRANKLIN DRUG CENTER
www.franklindrugcenter.com

FREEDOM DRUG
www.freedomdrug.com

HMI
www.inciid.org/hmi.html

IVP PHAMACEUTICAL CARE, INC
www.ivpcare.com (great music to listen to while browsing!)

POET'S PHARMACY
www.poetsrx.com

SCHRAFT'S PHARMACY
www.media-ware.com/schrafts

STOKE'S PHARMACY
www.stokesrx.com

SUPER VALUE HERBAL PHARMACY
www.super-value.com/homepage.htm

LARRY'S PHARMACY
www.liberty.com/home/foxfire

VILLAGE PHARMACY
members.aol.com/rxvillage/index.html

INTERNATIONAL

PROJECT ANFAP
www.ring.net/anfap/infert.htm

PHAMA-MED, LTD
www.pmed.com

SURROGACY & EGG DONATION

CALIFORNIA
Beverly Hills
Center for Surrogacy & Egg Donation, Inc.
www.eggdonor.com or
www.surroparenting.com

Garden Grove
Options National Registry
www.fertilityoptions.com
(also provides sperm and embryo donation)

Laguna Niguel
Surrogate Parenting Services
surrogateparenting.com

Walnut Creek
Family Fertility Center
www.surromother.com

COLORADO
Denver
Creating Families, Inc.
www.creatfam.com

GEORGIA
Marietta
The American Surrogacy Center
www.surrogacy.com

INDIANA
Indianapolis
Infertility Center of America
www.nkeane.com/ica/

Monrovia
Surrogate Mothers, Inc.
www.surrogatemothers.com

KENTUCKY
Louisville
Surrogate Parenting, Inc.
www.babies-by-levin.com

TEXAS
Austin
Surrogate Parenting Center of Texas
www.surrogacyagency.com

SPERM BANKS

CALIFORNIA

California Cryobank, Inc.
www.cryobank.com

Van Nuys

ZyGen Laboratories
www.zygen.com

Santa Anna & San Diego

The Fertility Center of California
www.fertilityctr.com

COLORADO

Loveland

CryoGam Colorado, Inc.
www.cryogam.com

FLORIDA

Altamonte Springs

United States Cryobanks of Florida
www.uscryo.com/sperm.html

MINNESOTA

Roseville

Cryogenic Laboratories, Inc.
www.cryolab.com

VIRGINIA

Fairfax

Fairfax Cryobank
www.givf.com/cryo1.html

OTHER ON-LINE BANKS

Xytex
www.mindspring.com/~xytex

APPENDIX C
SEARCHING TOOLS - WEB PAGES

DIRECTORIES

Yahoo

www.yahoo.com

AND is boolean operator used on multiple word queries, when not specified
➡ Automatically puts a wild card after every word (surroga ' surrogate ' surrogacy)
➡ Availability to conduct same search from multiple search engines at bottom of page

NetGuide Live

www.netguide.com

Look Smart

www.looksmart.com

Magellan

www.mckinley.com

OR is boolean operator used on multiple word queries, when not specified
➡ AND, OR, AND NOT boolean operators available
➡ Parentheses can be used to nest complex queries (embryo AND (adoption OR donation))
➡ "+" or "-" symbols can be used with words which must or must not appear in document

PointCom

www.pointcom.com

Web 411

www.sserv.com/web411

Nerd World

www.nerdworld.com

SEARCH ENGINES

Infoseek

www.infoseek.com

AND is boolean operator used on multiple word queries, when not specified
➡Quotes can be used to find phrases (ie "embryo adoption")
➡"+" or "-" symbols can be used with words which must or must not appear in document

Lycos

www.lycos.com
OR is boolean operator used on multiple word queries, when not specified
➡AND boolean operator available
➡"-" symbol can be used with words which must not appear in document
➡"$" symbol can be use for inclusive matches (fertil$ ' fertility, fertile)

HotBot

www.hotbot.com
AND, OR boolean operators available
➡Can also search by media type (Acrobat, Java, i.e. extension type)
➡ "-" symbol can be used with words which must not appear in document
➡Parentheses can be used to nest complex queries (embryo AND (adoption OR donation))

Webcrawler

www.webcrawler.com
OR is boolean operator used on multiple word queries, when not specified
➡AND, OR, NOT, NEAR, ADJ boolean operators available
➡ADJ term must appear next to each other in order (embryo ADJ adoption)
➡Quotes can be used to find phrases (ie "embryo adoption")

AltaVista

altavista.digital.com
Case INsensitive, (ie. FERTILITY ' Fertility ' fertility)
➡Quotes can be used to find phrases (ie "embryo adoption")
  AND, OR, NEAR, AND NOT boolean operators available
➡"+" or "-" symbols can be used with words which must or must not appear in document
➡Parentheses can be used to nest complex queries (embryo AND (adoption OR donation))

Excite

www.excite.com
OR is boolean operator used on multiple word queries, when not specified
➡AND, OR, AND NOT boolean operators available
➡"+" or "-" symbols can be used with words which must or must not appear in document
➡Parentheses can be used to nest complex queries (embryo AND (adoption OR donation))

166

Open Text

index.opentext.com
AND is boolean operator used on multiple word queries, when not specified
➡ AND, OR, NEAR, BUT NOT, FOLLOWED BY boolean operators available

World Wide Web Worm

wwww.cs.colorado.edu/wwww
AND is boolean operator used on multiple word queries, when not specified
➡ OR boolean operator available

META SEARCH ENGINES

Metacrawler

www.metacrawler.com
Searches 9 engines
➡ AND, OR, NEAR boolean operators available
➡ Ranks returns by confidence level

Search.com

www.search.com

Highway 61

www.highway61.com
Searches 7 engines
➡ Ranks results by confidence level, independent of who's search engine it is
➡ AND, OR boolean operators available

SavvySearch

guaraldi.cs.colostate.edu:2000/form
Searches 28 sources
➡ Multi-language capabilities

GUIDED TOURS

BabyZone℠

www.babyzone.com
Site exclusively covers pregnancy, childbirth, and infertility Web page reviews

The Mining Company

www.miningco.com

WEB PAGES LISTING SEARCH ENGINES

All-In-One

www.albany.net/allinone

Beaucoup

www.beaucoup.com/engines.html
Over 600 search tools listed
Publishes a FREE search magazine

SEARCHING TOOLS - NEWSGROUPS

Deja News

www.dejanews.com

Reference.COM

www.reference.com

ALSO:

AltaVista

altavista.digital.com

Excite

www.excite.com

HotBot

www.hotbot.com

Infoseek

www.infoseek.com

SUGGESTED READING

Fertility Books

Your Fertility Signals: Using Them to Achieve or Avoid Pregnancy Naturally, by Merryl Winstein (Smooth Stone Press, 1991)

Taking Charge of Your Fertility: The Definitive Guide to Natural Birth Control and Pregnancy Achievement, by Toni Weschler, MPH (Harperperennial Library, 1995)

Natural Fertility Awareness, by John & Lucie Davidson (Beckman Publishing, Inc., 1988)

Overcoming Infertility Naturally, by Karen Bradstreet (Woodland Publishers, 1994)

Herbal Remedies for Women: Discover Nature's Wonderful Secrets Just for Women, by Amanda McQuade Craford, M.N.I.M.H (Prima Press, 1997)

Herbal Healing for Women: Simple Home Remedies for Women of All Ages, by Rosemary Gladstar, Anna Vojtech (Fireside, 1993)

The Complete Woman's Herbal: A Manual of Healing Herbs and Nutrition for Personal Well-Being and Family Care, by Anne McIntyre (Henry Holt, 1994)

The Language of Fertility: A Revolutionary Mind-Body Program for Conscious Conception, by Niravi B Payne, MS and Brenda Lane Richardson (Random House, 1997)

Taking Charge of Infertility, by Patricia Johnston (Perspectives Press, 1995)

How to Be a Successful Fertility Patient: Your Guide to Getting the Best Possible Medical Help to Have a Baby, by Peggy Robin (Quill, 1993)

The Infertility Maze: Finding Your Way to the Right Help and the Right Answers, by Kassie Schwan (Contemporary Books, 1988)

Beyond Second Opinions: Rethinking Questions About Fertility, by Judith Steinberg Turiel (California Press, 1997)

The Fertility Sourcebook: Everything You Need To Know, by M. Sara Rosenthal (Contemporary Books, 1996)

Surviving Infertility: A Compassionate Guide Through the Emotional Crisis of Infertility, by Linda P. Salzer (Harper Collins, 1996)

Getting Pregnant When You Thought You Couldn't: The Interactive Guide That Helps You Up the Odds, by Helane S. Rosenberg, PhD, and Yakov M. Epstein, PhD (Warner Books, 1993)

Sweet Grapes: How to Stop Being Infertile and Start Living Again, by Jean W. Carter, PhD and Michael Carter (Perspectives Press, 1991)

Understanding Infertility: Insights for Family and Friends, by Patricia Irwin Johnston (Perspectives Press, 1997)

How Can I Help? : A Handbook of Practical Suggestions for Family and Friends of Couples Going Through Infertility, by Merle Bobmardieri, LICSW and Diane Clapp, BSN, RN (Wellspring Publications, Lexington, MA)

How to Become Your Own Best Infertility Counselor: Helping You Understand Your Struggle; Deciding What's Best for You and Educating Others to Accept, by Joyce Sutkamp Friedeman, PhD, CS, LPCC (Jolance Press, 1996)

Dr. Richard Marrs' Fertility Book: America's Leading Infertility Expert Tells You Everything You Need to Know About Getting Pregnant, by Richard Marrs, MD, Lisa Friedman Bloch, and Kathy Kirtland Silverman (Dell Books, 1998)

Infertility: Your Questions Answered, by S.L. Tan, MD, Howard S. Jacobs, MD, and Machelle M Seiber, MD (Birch Lane Press, 1995)

Overcoming Infertility: A Compassionate Resource for Getting Pregnant, by Robert Jansen, MD (W H Freeman & Co., 1997)

The Couple's Guide to Fertility: How New Medical Advances Can Help You Have a Baby, Gary Berger, MD, Marc Goldstein, MD, and Mark Fuerst (Doubleday, 1989)

The Infertility Book: A Comprehensive Medical & Emotional Guide, by Carla Harkness (Celestial Arts, 1992)

Getting Pregnant!, by Melvin J. Frisch, MD, and Gayle Rapoport (Hp Books, 1987)

Infertility: The Emotional Journey, by Michelle Fryer Hanson (Fairview Press, 1994)

Healing Mind, Healthy Woman: Using the Mind-Body Connection to Manage Stress and Take Control of Your Life, by Alice Domar and Henry Dreher (Delta, 1997)

Preventing Miscarriage: The Good News, by Jonathan Scher, MD, Carol Dix (Harper Collins, 1991)

Our Stories of Miscarriage: Healing with Words, edited by Karen Fitton and Rachel Faldet (Fairview Press, 1997)

The Ache for a Child, by Debra Bridwell (Chariot Victor Books, 1994)

Long-Awaited Stork: A Guide to Parenting After Infertility, by Ellen Sarasohn Glazer (Jossey-Bass Publishers, 1998)

While Waiting, by George E. Verrilli, M.D., F.A.C.O.G. and Anne Marie Mueser, Ed. D. (St. Martins Press, 1993)

Your Pregnancy Week-by-Week, by Glade B. Curtis, M.D., F.A.C.O.G. (Fisher Books, 1997)

Pregnant Fathers: Becoming the Father You Want to Be, by Jack Heinowitz, Ph.D. (Andrews & McMeel, 1997)

A Child Is Born, by Lennart Nilsson (Delta, 1994)

The Pregnancy Journal: A Day-By-Day Guide With Practical Information and Helpful Advice for a Healthy Pregnancy, by A. Christine Harris, Ph.D. (Chronicle Books, 1996)

What to Expect When You're Expecting, by Arlene Eisenberg, Heidi E. Murkoff, and Sandee E. Hathaway, B.S.N. (Workman Publishing Company, 1991)

Internet Books

Teach Yourself the Internet in 24 Hours, by Noel Estabrook, Sams Publishing, (1997)

Net.Search: Quickly Find Anything You Need on the Internet, by William Eager, Larry Donahue, Davide Forsyth, Kenneth Mitton, and Martin Waterhouse, Que Education & Training, (1995)

101 Essential Tips Using the Internet, by Chris Lewis, Dorling-Kindersley Ltd, London, (1997)

The Complete Indiot's Guide to the Internet, by Peter Kent, Que Education & Training, (1996)

The Internet for Dummies Quick Reference, by John R. Levine, Margaret Levine Young, & Arnold Reinhold, IDG Books Worldwide, (1997)

Index

OTHER BOOKS FROM CONCEIVING CONCEPTS

Are *You* Wishing for a Baby?
Now get the best resource to help manage your fertility!

This beautiful spiral-bound workbook contains 10 sections to help manage the emotions (and often treatment) in undertaking this life-changing event. Each tabbed section contains a guide to the subject, along with suggested reading and Web sites.

Topics include:

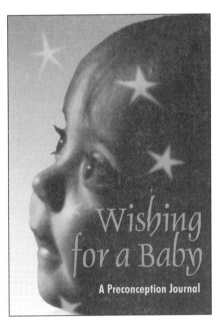

- Charting your Fertility Signs (organized charts to help record your BBT, cervical fluid & position, and many, many, more signs!)
- Daydreaming of Your Child (space to write to your future child!)
- Natural Fertility Treatments (record any treatments, practices you are undertaking)
- Fertility Decision Making (10 questions to answer every time you need to make a decision regarding entering, continuing, or ending treatment)
- Managing Friends & Family (practice great comeback lines)
- Medical Fertility Intervention (record all the test results which are conducted!)
- Doctor's Appointments (record what's said, and questions to ask at your next appointment)
- Grief/Pregnancy Loss (write down the emotions of your loss)
- Money, Money, Money (record all the money you've spent trying for that bundle of joy!)
- Success! (record how you found out, told your spouse, hormone levels, and ultrasound findings!)

Available at bookstores, or order from our Internet site located at:
www.conceivingconcepts.com

TIRED OF BOOKMARKING ALL THE SITES IN THIS BOOK? ARE YOU MISSING ANY NEW SITES?

NOW YOU DON'T HAVE TO!

Order your disk copy or subscription to *Infertility on the Internet* on an easy-to-use bookmarked diskette! All of the 250 sites featured in this book - PLUS over 50 new sites!

OR – order a one year subscription of the diskette – updated quarterly!

Description	Unit Price	Quantity	Total Price
Infertility on the Internet – the book*	$14.95	_____	_____
Bookmarked sites on 3 ½ inch diskette**	$6.95	_____	_____
1 year subscription on diskette**	$18.95	_____	_____
		Subtotal	_____
		Tax (KY Residents add 6% sales tax)	_____
		Shipping & Handling - add $3 per book	_____
		TOTAL	_____

*   Discounts available for volume orders. Call Conceiving Concepts at (502) 241-8497
** Shipping & Handling included in diskette price

Send check or money order (US dollars) with this form to:

Conceiving Concepts, Inc.
PO Box 869
Crestwood, KY 40014

Or call us at (502) 241-8497
with your Visa/Mastercard number to place your order.